Too Poor To Be Sick
Access to Medical Care for the Uninsured

Too Poor To Be Sick

Access to Medical Care for the Uninsured

Patricia A. Butler, JD

APHA Public Health Policy Series

American Public Health Association
1015 Fifteenth Street, NW
Washington, DC 20005

American Public Health Association
1015 Fifteenth Street, NW
Washington, DC 20005

William H. McBeath, MD, MPH, Executive Director

The opinions expressed in this publication are the author's and do not necessarily represent the views or official policies of the Association.

ISBN 0-87553-151-2
1M8/88; 1M6/89

Printed in the United States of America

Composition: Action Comp Co., Inc., Baltimore, Maryland
Set in: Century Expanded, Avant Garde Demi
Printing and binding: St. Mary's Press, Hollywood, Maryland
Cover design: Dan Winter, Emerson Braxton & Co., Silver Spring, Maryland

This book is dedicated to the memory of Beverlee A. Myers, whose tireless commitment to the goal of equitable access to health care for all Americans inspires us to continue pursuing that elusive but vital objective.

Contents

Appreciation is extended to Alan Monheit, National Center for Health Services Research, for new data analysis, and to Randy Desonia, Judy Glazner, Dianne Rowland, and Katherine Swartz for their careful reviews and thoughtful comments.

Preface

In 1986 more than a million Americans reported that they had tried to obtain needed health care but were unable to do so because of its cost. Several million more reported that financial barriers had made it difficult to acquire necessary medical services. A large number of particularly vulnerable populations, such as pregnant women and the chronically ill, fail to receive medical supervision of their conditions. Despite a federal law protecting emergency room patients from precipitous transfers, scandalous examples of such patient "dumping" persist. Although geographic, cultural, and educational barriers impede access to medical services, cost is the primary obstacle to receiving primary care. People who are poor, especially those without public or private insurance, face particular hurdles in obtaining health care services; this problem is compounded by the fact that the health of poor people is worse overall than the general population, thus increasing their need for care. Even higher income families can experience access problems if their insurance is inadequate. Such barriers to access have consequences in both human and economic terms: Millions of people forego entirely or delay seeking primary care until their need for treatment becomes urgent and then turn to hospital emergency rooms, which are legally obligated to treat them. These people experience increased suffering, and because they are in later stages of illness, their treatment is more costly.

The problem of access to medical care has increased in the United States over the last decade because of the convergence of three trends: an apparent growth in the number of Americans without public or private health insurance; the rise in the price of medical care, which has increased more rapidly than inflation, making even primary care less affordable to uninsured families and especially the poor; and the price competition among hospitals and other health care providers, which limits the cross-subsidies among payers through which charity care has traditionally been financed.

Many of the uninsured poor are eligible to receive medical care through a potpourri of state and local health care financing and delivery approaches. Medicaid is the best known of these financing programs. But almost all states and most local governments also finance and/or deliver health care to the poor who are not eligible for Medicaid, through funding public hospitals and clinics and through Medicaid-like programs that entitle eligible residents to obtain care from private sector physicians and hospitals. Over the past 5 years, state and local governments have begun to reexamine systematically this patchwork of public programs to determine how better to meet a growing need with static or shrinking revenues.

From these analyses has come an impressive variety of state strategies for indigent care that run the gamut from modest to comprehensive and incremental to universal. For instance, a few states have augmented primary care for pregnant women and children, and many states have expanded their Medicaid programs to cover additional eligible groups and capitalize on federal financial sharing. Some states are experimenting with small-scale projects to increase opportunities for the working poor to buy health insurance, and, as we went to press, Massachusetts had enacted strong incentives for most employers in the state to offer insurance to their workers. States are also exploring new means of financing health care programs for indigent people, such as taxing health care providers and alcohol and tobacco taxes.

These state and local initiatives are commendable and should be encouraged, because in addition to meeting specific and pressing current needs, they permit local demonstration of myriad approaches to financing and delivering care, targeting resources, managing cost and utilization, assuring quality, and raising revenue. These state experiences can serve as models for a broader national health care financing program.

Ultimately, however, the problem of access to medical care for all Americans is a national one that must be addressed at the federal level. This is true partly because federal tax, pension, and Medicaid laws impair the states' ability to craft the most comprehensive and appropriate health care financing programs to meet their needs. But more important, if medical care is recognized as a human good, not a market commodity, the nation is obliged to secure for all residents access to basic medical services, a step that many states are unlikely to take because of limited resources and political viewpoints. By failing to adopt an explicit federal policy of access to health care, we have sanctioned an implicit one: tax-subsidized private insurance for middle- and upper-class families, a publicly financed program for many of the poor, but no basic medical care financing protection for about half of the very poor and millions of near poor.

Just as current state efforts range from the nominal to the comprehensive, a modest federal health care access policy could be designed by refining current income tax, pension, and Medicaid and Medicare laws. Such changes would increase financing for care for many of the poor or uninsured, but only a comprehensive federal policy that directly increases the current means for financing medical services is likely to solve the nation's health care access problem. Several such approaches are currently under discussion in Congress, including requiring employers to offer health insurance to workers, providing financial assistance to marginally profitable employers, and publicly funded programs for the unemployed. An alternative strategy, drawn from the Canadian experience, would be a federal mandate that all states assure that their residents have health insurance or other financing protection that meets minimum national standards. These programs would be financed jointly with state and federal funds, with the formula based on a state's ability to raise revenues. A federalized model would allow states flexibility to determine whether to establish purely public programs or a mix of public and private health care financing strategies.

The design features of any national health care program raise numerous issues, but we should not now become paralyzed by such details. Rather, we must reach a political consensus on the basic principle that access to medical care is a national problem that compels a national solution. The 1988 presidential election campaign provides a propitious opportunity to place the health care access policy issue on the national political agenda. In anticipating a new national administration in 1989, it is imperative to make access to basic health care for all Americans the highest priority for serious congressional and executive attention.

Patricia A. Butler
August 1988

1

The Problem of Access
to Medical Care

The United States faces a serious and worsening problem that requires a national solution—the decreasing ability of many of its citizens to obtain needed medical care. Millions of Americans report having trouble obtaining medical care because of its cost. By even the most objective standards, many children, pregnant women, and chronically ill people do not receive necessary routine primary care. Access to care is an issue that has increased in significance in the 1980s because of reductions in Medicaid coverage of the poor, the growing number of people without private health insurance, conscious policies of many private hospitals to limit charity care despite expanding need in order to be price competitive, and the inability of public facilities to meet the growing demand. The policy issue posed by these converging forces is how to meet the long-standing societal responsibility to provide medical care for the poor in the face of both recent changes in employment patterns that limit access to health insurance and demands that the medical marketplace operate to lower prices and stem rising medical care expenditures.

This monograph explores the issue by describing (1) how many Americans experience difficulty obtaining medical care and why, (2) traditional means of financing and providing care to this population, (3) new state approaches to meet this growing need, and (4) a proposed national policy for addressing the problem on a broad

scale. This discussion should especially benefit state and local officials who are trying to meet the increasing needs of the uninsured,
but it is also timely and relevant to national debates about expanding national programs and increasing the federal role in assuring
access to medical care for the poor.

This monograph presents a spectrum of policy options to address the issue of access. These proposals are framed as a national
agenda because the poor, uninsured, and underinsured pose a national problem. Some proposed solutions acknowledge the importance—both political and practical—of federalism. A national
agenda could, for instance, give states discretion to design solutions that respond to unique local or regional differences in need,
demography, and economics. However, because the nation's problem of access to medical care has been accurately called "a national
disgrace (p. 26),"[1] it calls for a national remedy.

Congress considered a national program of medical care protection more than 40 years ago and enacted two components of such a
plan—Medicare and Medicaid—20 years ago. National health insurance was also under serious discussion 10 years ago, but concerns
about medical care expenditures stifled the deliberations.[2] It is appropriate that the question of access to medical care return to the
national agenda. This subject has reappeared in public debate with
increasing regularity, and the time is nearing when the nation will
confront the need to adopt an explicit national strategy to assure
that all Americans can obtain basic medical care.

This chapter defines and describes the problem of access to
medical care. The first section examines barriers to obtaining medical care, especially primary care. Focusing on financial impediments, the next three sections explore characteristics of the population without health insurance or with inadequate insurance,
emphasizing the particular burdens created by the combination of
poverty and lack of insurance. The fifth section discusses how current pressures to curb medical care spending by increasing price
competition affect hospital access for the poor and uninsured. The
final section is a summary that quantifies the extent of the unmet
need for medical care in the United States.

Why Access to Medical Care Is a Problem

Concerns about affordability and access to medical care have
surfaced recently in discussions at the national, state, and local lev-

els. The diverse parties in these debates characterize the problem variously as financing medical care for the poor, uncompensated hospital care, financing care for the uninsured, catastrophic medical care costs, or uncovered costs of caring for the elderly. This monograph defines the issue broadly as one of assuring access to primary care for all Americans. The focus is on access because many Americans, especially but not exclusively the poor, experience difficulty in obtaining medical care.[3] Thus, how to pay for the charity care provided by physicians and hospitals is an important but subordinate concern. The focus is on primary care because of its demonstrated contribution to improving health status.[4,5] The population under consideration is Americans at all income levels because although the poor, especially those without health insurance, face particular difficulty obtaining care, even higher income families can be financially devastated by a serious illness if they are uninsured or inadequately insured.[6]

Hospitals requesting financial relief from charity care and bad debt burdens often characterize the issue of medical care access as one of "uncompensated care."[7] Although a public policy to assist the poor, uninsured, and underinsured in obtaining medical care must also pay for that care, describing the problem as uncompensated care raises several problems. First, providers define uncompensated care in various ways. They may include not only charity to poor, uninsured patients, but also bad debt, which may be uncollectibles from people able, as well as those unable, to pay. They may also include discounts to private insurers and government payers. Second, some policy makers challenge the moves to bail out hospitals serving the poor as pouring increasing resources into inefficiently managed facilities and encouraging use of the most expensive primary care settings (hospital emergency rooms and outpatient departments). Finally, if the problem is seen as uncompensated care and its solution as paying hospitals for charity service, the poor who lack access to outpatient care will be hospitalized for conditions that could have been treated more cheaply and humanely with earlier interventions.

Given limitations on public resources, funding primarily hospital care, no matter how well intentioned, limits dollars for preventive and primary care programs, many of which are effective and can save long-term expenditures. Funding institutions may also force patients to use centralized facilities that are distant from home. Thus, the primary objective of programs for the poor and uninsured should not be to benefit medical care providers. The policy dilemma, however, is that the public and inner-city institutions serving the poor are less able to compete for private patients in the new medical care marketplace. Because these hospitals remain important last-resort providers of care to the poor and are often valuable community teaching and research facilities as well, one can justify explicit subsidies to assure their existence. But the tension persists between securing their survival and funding indigent care with limited resources.

The problem of care for the poor and the uninsured should be viewed as assuring individuals' access to care, not protecting institutions or practitioners. Considering established patterns of medical care use, it is likely that if the poor have better financial access many will continue to use public and teaching hospitals. Thus, a strategy focusing on financing care for individuals instead of financing institutions will continue to support these hospitals. But the problem will be appropriately defined as one of access, not institutional security.

Barriers to Access

Some policy makers ask for direct evidence of access barriers—examples of people unable to obtain needed medical care. Although the press has reported a few such instances,[8,9,10] the American medical care system generally provides emergency and urgent care for people who persistently seek it. Almost anyone presenting at a hospital emergency room, for instance, is treated and admitted, if necessary. A more subtle and pervasive problem, however, is the difficulty of obtaining appropriately early care, such as prenatal care or routine surveillance of chronic illness, without which subsequent treatment is more costly and often less effective.

Access to medical care can be measured subjectively and objectively. Subjective measures include individuals' perceptions of whether they have faced difficulty obtaining care or whether serious illness has been a financial hardship.[11] Because these indicators depend on respondents' understanding of their own health status and the utility of seeking medical care, they are not exclusive measures. But they are particularly useful for comparing perceptions of subgroups and for tracking trends over time. More objective measures of access to medical care include patterns of utilization, such as whether a person has a usual source of medical care, the frequency of physician or hospital visits, whether medical care meets an objective standard of need, or whether a person has received routine screening and treatment.[11,12] For some of these measures, such as immunizations or need for physician services for certain conditions, there is relative agreement on the appropriate frequency of care. For others, however, such as the number of physician visits per year for average adults, there may be no consensus. Thus, although such objective indicators may show disparities among groups, they do not fully establish which groups are receiving optimum amounts of health care. In combination, however, subjective and objective measures can provide a rough picture of the extent to which Americans appear to need and obtain medical care.

Comprehensive national surveys of medical care access in 1976 and 1982* found that by objective measures of third-party insurance coverage and physician and hospital contacts (both total numbers and those adjusted for certain indicators of need), the poor had continued over 30 years to close the gap with higher income groups:[11,12] In 1982 the poor were still less likely than higher income groups to use physician services, however.[13] The poor, people enrolled in public programs, and the uninsured all increased routine preventive care (annual blood pressure readings, pap smears, and breast examinations) between 1976 and 1982, but their use remained below both national averages and those of the higher income and privately insured populations.[11] In 1982 the low-income and the uninsured groups were also more likely than others to report difficulty in obtaining care (families for which serious illness caused financial problems, that needed help but did not get it, and those refused care).[11]

---

*The 1976 survey involved in-person interviews, whereas the 1982 survey was conducted by telephone (which may have biased results against rural and poor people, who are less likely than urban and higher-income people to have phones). Although analysts made comparisons between the surveys only when questions were "similar,"[11] the different survey methods may have elicited different responses. Consequently, comparisons must be seen as approximate but are the best data available.

A 1986 national survey asked different questions about access but reached similar conclusions.* Sixteen percent of Americans (about 39 million) reported needing medical care but having difficulty obtaining it, half of them for financial reasons.[3] About 1 million people (0.4%) reported that they tried to get care but could not because of cost.[3] Among people with serious or chronic conditions (such as heart disease, cancer, diabetes, hypertension, or stroke), 17% had not visited a physician during the year, although it is generally agreed that they should have at least one such visit a year.[13] The poor, blacks, and Hispanics with these conditions were somewhat less likely than Americans as a whole to visit physicians. Although early prenatal care is well recognized to be cost-effective,[14] 15% of all pregnant women had not received first-trimester care; the poor were twice as likely as all Americans not to have received it, and the uninsured were somewhat more likely than all Americans not to have received it.[13] Hypertension is an asymptomatic illness that when uncontrolled can be costly in human and economic terms.[15] In 1986, 20% of all Americans with known hypertension had no high blood pressure check. For this measure, the poor were somewhat better off than average, but blacks and Hispanics were less likely than other groups to have had such screening.[13]

These 1986 data also show that only 82% of Americans have a usual source of health care. Such a contact point is important because patients can receive more appropriate, timely, and effective medical care if they have a single place where they can go regularly for care.[13] The uninsured, the poor, Hispanics, blacks, and the chronically ill were much more likely than other Americans to be without a usual source of care in 1986.[3]

Geographic, cultural, and racial factors contribute to problems of access. For instance, a disproportionate number of people who are in fair or poor health and have chronic illnesses live in rural areas,[3] where medical care is more difficult to obtain than in cities (although the differences in utilization between rural and urban residents appear to be declining).[13] Cultural traditions, such as a preference for home treatments or fear of medical practitioners, as

---

*The 1986 survey was conducted by telephone, with additional in-person interviews of people without telephones. The survey found significantly fewer uninsured people than Current Population Surveys for the same year (9.0% vs. 15.7%), possibly because of differences in methodology.[3] The 1986 survey data are, however, the most recent and best available to measure subjective and objective access barriers.

well as the difficulty of finding health professionals sensitive to cultural differences, influence decisions to seek care.[16] Racial discrimination is also believed responsible for minorities' less-than-average use of care despite greater-than-average need.[17] However, the primary discriminators between families with and without access are income* and health insurance coverage. The poor and uninsured are much more likely to experience both subjective and objective access problems than the nonpoor or the insured. Considering the substantial financial burden that even fairly small medical costs impose on the uninsured poor,[6] it is not surprising that the poor delay or forego preventive and routine primary care. Because poverty, lack of insurance, and inadequate insurance predict access problems, this chapter describes the relevant characteristics of these populations.

The Importance of Primary Care

The extent to which medical care contributes to improved health is sometimes questioned in debates on care for the poor and uninsured. Certainly, social, environmental, nutritional, and other life-style factors[18] are important influences on overall health status, but the evidence is clear that medical care does affect health. Primary care has been shown, for instance, to contribute to improved health in children by reducing neonatal mortality and by improving detection and control of congenital disease, diabetic ketoacidosis, asthma, teenage pregnancy, epilepsy, and rheumatic fever.[4] Part of the reduction in mortality rates for some conditions among adults, such as ischemic heart disease and cardiovascular diseases, has also been attributed to increased medical care.[5,19]

A particularly poignant illustration of the value of primary medical care to the chronically ill is a study of the effects of changes in Medicaid coverage in California. Indigent adults were removed from the state-funded Medicaid program and required to use county hospitals rather than their previous private physicians. Pa-

---

*National studies on health care access and use measure poverty by income and family size. They do not consider personal resources, which measure ability to pay for health care by using savings, liquidating assets, or borrowing funds. Although some near-poor and lower-middle-class families can pay for health care with their assets, other than the temporarily unemployed, very few poor families have significant savings or borrowing power. Thus, low-income status is an appropriate indicator of inability to pay for care.

tients with hypertension or diabetes received less medical supervision of these conditions and experienced a significant deterioration of health status measured by clinical examination and elevation of blood pressure, compared with a control group of Medicaid adults. Four of the five indigent adults who died during the study period had experienced financial barriers to care.[20]

The Population at Risk

People facing financial access barriers to medical care are often labeled "medically indigent," but this term is ambiguous. It is sometimes used to mean all the poor, but because Medicaid pays for medical care for a large share of the poor, its beneficiaries might not be properly classified as medically indigent. The term sometimes includes only people who are uninsured and poor, but this definition excludes middle-income families who have limited or no insurance and face catastrophic health care episodes. Although these higher income families can usually obtain routine ambulatory care, their economic security may be jeopardized when they need hospitalization or long-term rehabilitation services. For these reasons, this monograph does not refer to the "medically indigent." Rather, it describes and analyzes the financial barriers of lack of insurance, inadequate insurance, and poverty—the primary impediments to access to medical care.

Lack of Health Insurance

Although geographic, cultural, and racial factors may impede access to medical care, the existence of health insurance can significantly ameliorate differences in access among income groups. Over the past 10 years, research at the national and state levels has revealed changing health insurance coverage and a close relationship between insurance and use of medical care.

There are several sources of data on health insurance coverage. Those most often cited are the National Medical Care Expenditure Survey (NMCES) of 1977, the Census Bureau's annual Current Population Survey (CPS), and the Census Bureau's Quarterly Survey of Income and Program Participation (SIPP). These surveys cover different time periods, and, although they all include health insurance coverage and demographic data, only NMCES contains information on health status, health care use, and scope of insur-

Table 1.1—Uninsured Persons Under Age 65 in Millions
(and as a percentage of the U.S. population)

Survey	Year						
	1977	1980	1982	1983	1984	1985	1986
NMCES	26.2	—	—	—	—	—	—
	(13.8)	—	—	—	—	—	—
CPS	—	28.6	30.7	32.7	35.1	34.7	37.0
	—	(14.6)	(15.2)	(16.1)	(17.1)	(17.4)	(17.6)
SIPP	—	—	—	35.0	32.0	31.0	—
	—	—	—	(17.0)	(15.0)	(15.0)	—

Sources: NMCES and CPS data from Sulvetta MB, Swartz K. The uninsured and uncompensated care—A chart book. Washington, DC: National Health Policy Forum, George Washington University, 1986. SIPP data from U.S. Bureau of the Census.

ance. Researchers debate the relative merits of the various data sources, voicing particular concerns about the age of NMCES and the recall period of CPS. A more detailed description of the strengths and weaknesses of these data sources is presented in Appendix A.

Despite their differences, all three data sources can be used as a foundation for national and state policy. It may not be critical to pinpoint, for instance, the precise number of uninsured people. Establishing a range from several current sources may suffice. And although NMCES may not provide accurate estimates of current insurance coverage, it illustrates differences in patterns of use between the insured and uninsured,[21] differences that have been mirrored in more recent studies.[22]

Who Is Uninsured?

The number and proportion of Americans under age 65* without third-party coverage by either private insurance or public programs (Medicaid and Medicare) increased from 1980 through 1983 from 14.6% (28.6 million) to 16.1% (32.7 million) (Table 1.1). In the subsequent 3 years, according to CPS, the proportion of uninsured

---

*The population under age 65 is the focus of this section because almost all the elderly are covered by Medicare, and the worse health status and greater use patterns of the elderly insured can distort comparisons between insured and uninsured groups.

Table 1.2—Percentage of People Under Age 65 by Source of Health Insurance Coverage, 1983 and 1985

Source of Health Insurance	Year	
	1983	1985
Private coverage	75.7*	73.6*
Employer plan	67.1	65.1
Other plan	12.7	12.3
Public coverage	12.9	12.8
Medicaid	8.0	8.1
Medicare	2.3	2.2
CHAMPUS	3.3	3.1
No coverage	16.1	17.4

Source: U.S. Dept. of Commerce, Bureau of the Census.
*Percentages for categories of private coverage add up to more than totals because some people had coverage from more than one source.

has continued to rise slowly, but according to SIPP, it has declined and leveled off. Between 31 and 37 million people (15.0 to 17.6%) are currently uninsured, far above pre-recession levels.

The post-recession increase in the rate at which Americans are uninsured appears due primarily to declining private insurance coverage (Table 1.2). From 1983 to 1985, 2% of the privately insured (about 4 million people) lost coverage. This drop in private insurance appears to be attributable to a large extent to shifting patterns of employment—the substitution of jobs in small, service, and start-up firms, which frequently do not offer health insurance, for those in larger manufacturing firms, which were more likely to offer insurance. It may also be due to the increasing cost of health insurance premiums, which has caused some employers to drop insurance coverage or require employees to share in premium costs, which are unaffordable to many low-wage workers. Although the proportionate increase in the uninsured appears small, the trend contrasts with the steady post-war decline in the percentage of Americans without insurance.

Income. The uninsured are primarily the poor (Table 1.3). More than one-third of the uninsured in 1984 had incomes below the federal poverty level (about $10,000 for a family of four), and more than half had incomes below 150% of the poverty level. Furthermore, as shown in Table 1.4, the likelihood of being uninsured is

Table 1.3—Distribution of the Uninsured of All Ages by Income Level, 1984

Income Level	Percentage
Below poverty	35.6
1–1.49 times poverty	16.7
1.5–1.99 times poverty	12.6
2–2.99 times poverty	15.4
3 times poverty and above	19.7
Total	100.0

Source: Sulvetta MB, Swartz K. The uninsured and uncompensated care—A chart book. Washington, DC: National Health Policy Forum, George Washington University, 1986.

inversely related to income. It is interesting to note, however, that 15% of people who are uninsured have incomes between 200% and 300% of the poverty level, and almost 20% have incomes greater than 300% of the poverty level. These families can probably pay for routine primary medical care but may have difficulty affording the cost of hospitalization or a long-term chronic illness, especially if their assets are limited or nonliquid.

Age. Despite the existence of Medicaid coverage for many poor children, children under 18 years old constitute the largest age group among the uninsured. One-third of the uninsured are children under age 18, and nearly one-quarter are 18- to 24-year-olds (Table 1.5). More than 40% of these uninsured children live in families below the poverty level. The likelihood of being uninsured is greatest among 18- to 24-year-olds, who are often in college, graduate school, or entry level jobs without private insurance and who

Table 1.4—Percentage Uninsured Among People Under Age 65 by Income Level, 1984

Income Level	Percentage Uninsured
Below poverty	33.8
1–1.49 times poverty	24.7
1.5–1.99 times poverty	18.4
2–2.99 times poverty	11.6
3 times poverty and above	7.0

Source: Sulvetta MB, Swartz K. The uninsured and uncompensated care—A chart book. Washington, DC: National Health Policy Forum, George Washington University, 1986.

Table 1.5—Age Distribution of the Uninsured
Population Under Age 65, 1984

Age	Percentage
0–17	33.0
18–24	23.6
25–34	17.7
35–44	9.7
45–54	7.7
55–64	8.3
Total	100.0

Source: Sulvetta MB, Swartz K. The uninsured and uncompensated care—A chart book. Washington, DC: National Health Policy Forum, George Washington University, 1986.

may choose to be uninsured because they are relatively healthy (Table 1.6).

Race and Marital Status. Although most of the uninsured are white, minorities are at greater risk of being uninsured (Tables 1.7 and 1.8). Married women are more likely to be uninsured than married men, and women with spouses absent are much more likely to be uninsured than men with spouses absent. Divorced women and men are both about twice as likely as their married counterparts to be uninsured (Table 1.9). Among divorced people, lack of insurance may be felt most by women, who are likely both to require more medical care themselves and to have custody of young children who

Table 1.6—Percentage Uninsured Among
People Under Age 65 by Age, 1984

Age	Percentage Uninsured
0–17	18.6
18–24	29.0
25–34	15.4
35–44	11.3
45–54	12.0
55–64	13.0

Source: Sulvetta MB, Swartz K. The uninsured and uncompensated care—A chart book. Washington, DC: National Health Policy Forum, George Washington University, 1986.

Table 1.7—Racial Distribution of the Uninsured
Population Under Age 65, 1984

Race	Percentage Uninsured	
	Adults*	Children
White	79.3	76.0
Black	17.3	20.0
Other	3.5	4.0
Total	100.0	100.0

Source: Sulvetta MB, Swartz K. The uninsured and uncompensated care—A chart book. Washington, DC: National Health Policy Forum, George Washington University, 1986.
*Percentages add up to more than 100% because of rounding.

Table 1.8—Percentage Uninsured Among
People Under Age 65 by Racial Group, 1984

Race	Percentage Uninsured	
	Adults	Children
White	15.0	17.4
Black	25.0	24.6
Other	21.0	22.0

Source: Sulvetta MB, Swartz K. The uninsured and uncompensated care—A chart book. Washington, DC: National Health Policy Forum, George Washington University, 1986.

Table 1.9—Percentage Uninsured Among
People Under Age 65 by Marital Status, 1984

Marital Status	Percentage Uninsured	
	Men	Women
Married	9.7	10.5
Spouse absent	26.3	36.0
Widowed	17.7	21.5
Divorced	23.3	19.9
Separated	29.8	24.6
Never married	30.6	25.0

Source: Sulvetta MB, Swartz K. The uninsured and uncompensated care—A chart book. Washington, DC: National Health Policy Forum, George Washington University, 1986.

Table 1.10—Distribution of the Uninsured Under
Age 65 by Employment and Dependent
Category, 1980

Status	Percentage
Employed uninsured	55.6
Full-time	38.7
Part-time	16.9
Uninsured dependents of employed	22.3
Other uninsured	22.1*

Source: Monheit AC, Hagan MM, Berk ML, Farley PJ. The employed
uninsured and the role of public policy. Inquiry 1985;22:348–364.
*Includes 10–12% who are uninsured dependents of insured workers.

need access to early, preventive care and are probably also
uninsured.[23]

Location of Residence. In 1977, 17.6% of residents of rural communities (4.5 million persons) were uninsured, compared with
10.4% of residents of the nation's 16 largest Standard Metropolitan
Statistical Areas and 12.6% nationally.[24] This disparity reflects the
prevalence of agriculture, small employers, and lack of unionization
in rural America. The percentage of uninsured residents of rural
areas is likely to have risen since 1977 as the farm crisis has
accelerated.

Employment. The risk of being uninsured is greater for people
who are unemployed, seeking work, or unable to work than for people who are employed, but more than half of the uninsured are
adult workers (Table 1.10), two-thirds of whom work full-time and
one-third part-time. In addition, 22% of the uninsured are dependents of uninsured workers,[25] and 10 to 12% of the uninsured are
dependents of insured workers,* so about 87 to 89% of the uninsured population is attached to the work force.[25] Studies showing
the large extent to which the uninsured are employed have repu-
diated the common myth that workers are insured and the unemployed are not. To be sure, 85% of working Americans are insured
through the workplace,[25] and health insurance has become an expected fringe benefit of most jobs.

The fact that many workers are uninsured raises different policy problems than states would face were most uninsured people

*Personal communication, Alan Monheit, National Center for Health Services Research.

not employed. For instance, the recent federal requirement in the Consolidated Budget Reconciliation Act of 1985 (COBRA) (PL 99–272) that employment group insurance be extended for several months after employment terminates addresses a need for interim protection for workers between jobs. But such a mandate does not assist people who are unemployed in paying the full premium, including the former employer's share. Nor does it confront the greater and longer term problem of people employed in or laid off from firms that never offered health insurance coverage in the first place. The fact that many uninsured people are stable, long-term workers rather than temporarily unemployed or mentally or physically disabled suggests that states must develop different strategies for addressing the problem.

Firms in which the uninsured are employed tend to be small, pay low wages, are not unionized, and are primarily agricultural and construction firms.[25] This employment pattern is consistent with the educational characteristics of the uninsured: The people most likely to have no insurance are those who have not completed high school.[24] In 1977 almost half of the people employed in firms with 25 or fewer employees had no insurance, compared with only 7.7% employed in firms with 26 to 250, 2.2% in firms with 251 to 999, and less than 1% in firms of 1,000 or more.[26] The Small Business Administration has estimated that in 1985 only 39% of firms with fewer than 25 employees offered health insurance, compared with 86% of firms having more than 500 employees.[27]

Studies have shown that the small firms offering insurance are much more likely to have higher deductibles and coinsurance than larger firms,* so workers in these firms have greater exposure for out-of-pocket costs.[29] Even with some recently increased cost-sharing features in large firms, these wide differences are likely to persist. Furthermore, employment-based insurance coverage is declining slightly (Table 1.2). This change appears to be due to the

---

*Employment is the primary source of the most comprehensive coverage. NMCES found that employment-related insurance coverage provides much richer benefits than insurance purchased outside the workplace. For instance, although 87% of people with employment-related insurance had basic plus major medical coverage, only 39% of people with non-employment-related insurance had such broad coverage. Similarly, people with employment-related coverage were much more likely than those with other insurance to be covered for dental and vision care, prescription drugs, physician office visits, physical exams, and outpatient psychiatric care.[28]

Table 1.11—Percentage Uninsured Among
People of All Ages by Region, 1984

Region	Percentage Uninsured
Pacific	17.0
Mountain	19.2
West North-Central	13.0
West South-Central	20.2
East North-Central	12.0
East South-Central	16.7
New England	10.5
Middle Atlantic	12.5
South Atlantic	16.7

Source: Sulvetta MB, Swartz K. The uninsured and uncompensated care—A chart book. Washington, DC: National Health Policy Forum, George Washington University, 1986.

changing employment pattern from manufacturing to service industry jobs and to the elimination by some firms of health insurance coverage. In a Boulder County survey, for example, 8% of the firms that did not offer insurance at the time of the survey had done so in the previous 2 years.[30]

Regional Differences. NMCES and CPS both show general regional differences in insurance coverage: In 1984 about 20% of the residents of the West South-Central and Mountain states were uninsured, followed by about 17% of the residents of the East South-Central, South Atlantic, and Pacific states (Table 1.11). The Northeastern, Middle Atlantic, and North-Central states were less likely to have uninsured residents. These regional comparisons are elucidated by studies conducted by more than half the states since 1983.*[31] State and local governments have become increasingly interested in the problem of the uninsured poor, partly because of the potentially costly legal responsibility to finance medical care for this group. The results of these state surveys (Table 1.12) are consistent with the regional variations noted by CPS and NMCES.

---

*State studies have been conducted in a variety of ways. For instance, New Mexico's research was a mailed questionnaire, whereas Colorado's was an in-person household survey. Other states estimated the number of uninsured people by approximations from national data, adjusted when possible for known local characteristics. States generally defined insurance in the same way as the national studies, so despite some methodological variations, their results should be roughly comparable.

Table 1.12—Percentage of Uninsured People in
Selected States

State	Percentage Uninsured
Minnesota	8.0
Rhode Island	8.0
Colorado	18.7
New Mexico	21.0

Sources: Shreve D. Indigent care in Minnesota. In: Curtis R, ed. Access to care for the medically indigent: A resource document for state and local officials. Washington, DC: Academy for State and Local Government, 1985.

Rhode Island Department of Health. 1985 Rhode Island Health Insurance Survey. Providence, RI: Author, 1986.

Colorado Task Force on the Medically Indigent. Colorado's sick and uninsured—We can do better. Denver, CO: Piton Foundation, 1984.

Bureau of Business and Economic Research. Health care coverage and the medically indigent in New Mexico. Albuquerque, NM: University of New Mexico, 1984.

These differences are explained by diverse Medicaid programs—often more generous in the Northeast and Midwest, for instance—and different employment patterns—the greater number of small and nonunion firms in the South and West.

Most of the states have reported data from only one specific time, making trends difficult to establish. A few states, however, such as New York, have longer-term data on insurance coverage. Like the national CPS data, these state studies suggest a slow but steady decline in insurance coverage. For instance, although 87% of New Yorkers were insured in 1980, only 84% were insured in 1984.[32] Rhode Island residents also experienced a small decline in insurance coverage from 94% to 92% between 1972 and 1985.[33] State trends depend not only on employment levels but also on structural changes in employment. If, as is predicted, the Midwest and Northeast move from manufacturing, a well-insured industry, to service industries, which are less likely to offer insurance as a fringe benefit, state rates of uninsurance are likely to increase.

Health Status of the Uninsured

In 1977 about half (46%) of the U.S. population rated its health as "excellent," 39% rated it as "good," 11% as "fair," and only 4% as "poor."[24] The uninsured under age 65 are less healthy than the insured: 15% of these uninsured people reported fair or poor health compared with 11% of the insured.[34]

Use of Medical Care by the Uninsured

Uninsured people at all income levels use fewer medical care services than do people who are insured. For instance, while overall rates of preventive care, such as blood pressure readings for all adults and pap smears and breast examinations for women, increased from 1976 to 1982, rates of such preventive care for the uninsured declined.[11] Similarly, in 1977 the uninsured under age 65 had only two-thirds as many physician visits* as the insured and only half as many hospital days.[36]

Use rates are especially low for the uninsured who are sick, poor, or both. For instance, in 1977 insured people in fair or poor health had 6.9 annual physician visits, compared with 4.1 for uninsured people in fair or poor health, and the differences were even greater for blacks and residents of rural areas.[34]

For the poor, the average number of physician visits per year has increased in the past 50 years (Figure 1.1). Whereas the poor once had fewer physician visits per year than the nonpoor, the averages became comparable in the late 1960s, shortly after enactment of Medicaid. By 1970 the poor saw physicians more often than the nonpoor. When adjusted for the fact that health status of the poor is generally worse than that of the nonpoor, physician visits in 1981 were roughly comparable among income groups, although the gap between rich and poor appears to have widened in 1986.[13] But poor people who are uninsured are less likely to visit physicians than poor people who are insured. In 1983, among Colorado residents whose incomes were less than 150% of the federal poverty level, the uninsured were somewhat less likely than the insured to have had one visit in the previous 2 months (16.9% vs. 19.2%), and they were much less likely to have had two visits in that period (12.5% vs. 21.5%).[22]

Furthermore, Colorado's uninsured poor in fair or poor health were only two-thirds as likely as the insured with similar health status to have had two or more visits in the previous 2 months.[22] In

---

*Because about 12% of people insured through their employment were not insured for physician visits,[35] a small fraction of the insured should have been considered uninsured for purposes of this comparison, which would slightly increase this disparity.

Fig. 1.1—Number of physician visits per person per year for poor and nonpoor people, 1931–81.

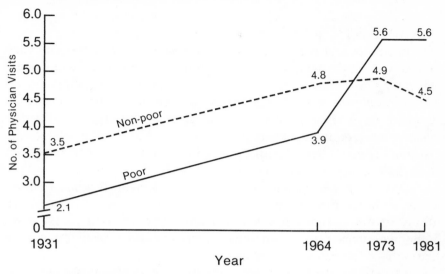

Source: Blendon R, Rogers D. Cutting medical care costs. JAMA 1983;250(1):1880–1885.

Copyright 1983, American Medical Association. Reprinted with permission.

1977, among people who were both poor (incomes less than 125% of the poverty level) and sick, the uninsured had only half as many physician visits and drug prescriptions and about two-thirds as many hospital days as those who were poor and sick but insured. These patterns persisted over various definitions of poor health status.[36] Similarly, children who were both poor and sick and who were eligible for Medicaid had almost as many physician contacts (9.3) as did middle-income children (10.0) in 1981, whereas children who were poor and sick but did not have Medicaid had fewer physician visits (7.7).[37]

Inadequate Insurance Coverage

Although policy makers have focused on the population without insurance as most likely to be unable to afford medical care, it is acknowledged that many people with insurance are not fully protected against the costs of needed medical care. A striking example of inadequate insurance is Medicare, which, because of increased cost sharing and limited coverage of long-term care and other services, has been estimated to cover only about 45% of the average health care bill of the elderly.*[38] Medicaid beneficiaries can also be underinsured: Some state programs do not cover many needed services (such as medical equipment, prosthetic devices, vision care, or dental care) and, because of payment limits and administrative problems, providers often refuse to participate in the program, leaving eligibles with an "entitlement" but no ready access to care.

Adequacy of health insurance is difficult to define precisely; it depends on the likelihood of needing medical care, the amount and cost of care required, specific policy limits, family size, and family income. Thus, underinsurance has no single definition. Using 1977 NMCES data on actual incidence of illness, family income, and insurance policy coverages, researchers have hypothesized several definitions of underinsurance and measured the magnitude of the underinsured population under each definition.[40] Because they examined only the population under age 65, the analysts did not evaluate the adequacy of Medicare coverage, but 1988 law expands Medicare to include protection from some catastrophic medical care costs, thus acknowledging the program's limitations.

For instance, if inadequate insurance is defined as having out-of-pocket costs exceeding 3% of family income, only about 5% of insured American families are inadequately insured. If, instead, the definition is a 1 in 20 chance that out-of-pocket expenses will exceed 10% of family income, about 8% of the population is underinsured. About 13% of the population is inadequately insured under a definition of a 1 in 100 chance that out-of-pocket expenses will exceed 10% of family income. If the definition is that there is no limit on the hospital costs for which an enrollee would be liable (ie, no "stop loss"), 40% of the population was underinsured in 1977 (estimated to be only 26% in 1984 due to improvements in coverage). Researchers estimate, therefore, that between 8 and 26% of the insured U.S. population is not adequately covered by its current insurance.[40]

By any of these definitions, women, dependents, the unemployed, the poor, people between 55 and 64 years of age, and people

---

*Some of the costs not covered by Medicare are paid by private insurance supplementary to Medicare and by Medicaid's payment of Medicare's cost sharing and nursing home care for the elderly poor. But two-thirds of the elderly below the federal poverty line are not covered by Medicaid, and they spend an average of 15% of their incomes on out-of-pocket medical expenses.[39]

with nongroup coverage are most likely to be underinsured. The underinsured are much more likely to report fair or poor health,[40] a finding consistent with the research model for actual use of health care: The likelihood of needing health care increases as health status declines. Combining data on the uninsured and the underinsured by various definitions, researchers have estimated that between 50 and 77 million people under age 65 are not protected by health insurance and may face either serious financial burdens or barriers in seeking medical care.[40]

The Financial Burden of Poverty and Lack of Insurance

Despite improvements in the past 20 years, the poor in America continue to have worse health status than higher income groups. It is unclear whether illness and disability cause poverty or vice versa, but the relationship is well recognized.[41,42] Thus, although infant mortality rates have dropped steadily since 1960, the rate among blacks (who are much more likely than whites to be poor[18]) in 1985 was still twice that of whites (18 deaths per 1,000 live births for blacks vs. 9 for whites).[43] Poor children are 75% more likely than higher income children to be admitted to a hospital in a given year, have 30% more restricted activity days and 40% more days lost from school due to illness, and suffer from more chronic conditions, such as anemia, blood lead, and asthma.[42] The 1986 national access survey found that low-income respondents were more than twice as likely as higher income respondents to report having fair or poor health.[13] Blacks and Hispanics were much more likely than whites to report having fair or poor health and chronic illness.[3]

The poor without insurance or with inadequate coverage are more likely to have worse health than other income groups[44] and are more likely to experience out-of-pocket medical expenses that are financially catastrophic.[6] Twenty percent of all American families (including people age 65 and over) had uninsured out-of-pocket medical care costs exceeding 5% of their annual income in 1977, the latest data available.[6] For about 10% of families, such costs exceeded 10% of their income, and for more than 4%, such costs exceeded 20% of their income.[6] Lower income families were, however, much more likely than higher income families to experience such proportionately high medical costs. In fact, almost one-third of families with incomes less than $12,000 in 1977 incurred out-of-pocket costs of at least 5% of their family income, compared with only 5% of families with annual incomes exceeding $20,000.[6]

These disparities remain when family size is taken into consideration. The likelihood of having uninsured medical expenses that exceeded 20% of income in 1977 was more than 10 times greater for families at or below the poverty level than for families with higher incomes.[6] The incomes of two-thirds of all families with such costs fell below the poverty level. The average expenditure for poverty level families was less than $1,000 in 1977, but this amount represented a large share of their annual incomes. The out-of-pocket costs of 70% of all families that incurred medical costs in excess of 20% of their income were under $2,000.[6]

These estimates are conservative, because they are based on 1977 data. Furthermore, they include only 1 year's expenditures, whereas catastrophic illness often lasts for 2 or 3 years.[45] Nor do the estimates include long-term nursing home care, which often bankrupts a family. The significant impact of out-of-pocket expenses between $1,000 and $2,000 on low-income families should be considered in designing any catastrophic insurance programs. Relatively low costs, such as the costs of preventive and routine care, can be a major burden for the poor.

Contribution of Medical Care Competition to the Access Problem

How Charity Care Is Financed

While the number of uninsured people has grown, their traditional sources of charity care have diminished. Many physicians have long provided some free and discounted care, but there is concern that the excess supply of physicians will increase competition and decrease physicians' incomes, thereby causing them to be less willing to maintain existing levels of charity, much less meet increased demands.[46] Community hospitals, primarily public and private nonprofit institutions, are also providers of both inpatient and ambulatory care to the poor and uninsured. As discussed in Chapter 2, hospital care for many of the poor is reimbursed by Medicaid and by state or local sources that fund public hospitals or provide grants to other hospitals serving the poor. But unsponsored care is financed primarily by implicit subsidies, the increased charges to paying patients—mostly those privately insured through Blue Cross, commercial carriers, or self-insured employers.

Market pressures have driven providers, especially hospitals, to become more competitive. Hospitals can compete in a number of ways—by emphasizing quality, specializing in unique services or those not covered by fee schedules, and cutting prices by cutting costs. Among the most obvious ways for most hospitals to compete is to limit charity care. Many states have long required hospitals with emergency rooms to treat all urgent patients regardless of payment source, and federal law now includes such a mandate. But hospitals have control over how much additional care they will provide. As discussed in Chapter 2, they are increasingly exercising their discretion in order to strike a balance between community responsibility and financial survival in the medical care market. Although total hospital charity care has grown slightly, the increase has come largely from public and inner-city hospitals, and the overall growth in hospital charity has not kept pace with the growth of the uninsured population.

Public hospitals are usually established with a charter to serve everyone, including the poor. In some parts of the country, inner cities are served by private nonprofit hospitals that effectively perform this same function. When the numbers of uninsured increase and most private hospitals limit their charity service, the public and inner-city hospitals experience greater demand.[9] Because government contributions to these institutions have not met growing need, such hospitals face conflicting pressures in the competitive health care marketplace. Need for their services has expanded but their income from private insurance, by which they subsidize unsponsored care, has declined.[47] Thus, the policy problem of access to medical care encompasses a concern for the survival of the institutions historically designed to serve the uninsured.

The Competitive Medical Marketplace

Public and private purchasers of health care have deemed unacceptable the inflation rate of medical care prices (7.5% in 1986, down from 11.6% in 1982), the growth in per capita medical care expenditures (increasing 9.8% from 1984 to 1985), and the increase of the percentage of the nation's gross national product devoted to health (up from 9.1% in 1980 to 10.7% in 1985).[48] Growing per capita medical care costs hit the poor directly, because without insurance, care is increasingly less affordable, and indirectly, because this growth has reduced the willingness and ability of the public and private sectors to continue to subsidize medical care for the poor.

Although states with hospital price regulation seem to have curbed the rate at which hospital costs are increasing,[49] the prevailing approach for reducing medical care expenditures is to encourage the medical care industry to act more like a traditional competitive economic market. Policy makers are eliminating many barriers to competition, such as restrictions on advertising and bed supply, and both government and private sector purchasers are trying to bargain with medical care providers for lower prices. Federal and state governments, which buy care for their employees as well as for Medicare, Medicaid, and other public beneficiaries, are beginning to expect hospitals and physicians to share in the financial risk of medical care through arrangements such as health maintenance organizations (HMOs). They are also setting physician and hospital prices in advance, instead of paying all incurred costs after service is rendered. And they are monitoring the cost and quality of care through peer review and utilization review organizations. Employers, who buy medical care indirectly through insurance and directly if they self-insure, are using the same techniques—risk sharing with providers, prospective payment, fee setting, and utilization review. Providers have responded to these demands at least in part because of the excess supply of physicians and hospital beds. This excess has created a medical care buyer's market in most areas of the country.

The wisdom of letting competition lower prices is well debated elsewhere.[49,50,51] The relevance of competition to this treatise, however, is that as medical care providers offer price discounts to meet marketplace expectations, they cut costs, including the implicit cost of charity care, much of which has traditionally provided needed inpatient and outpatient services for the poor. Some business leaders, recognizing that their pressures on hospitals to lower prices have encouraged reduction in care to the poor and uninsured, have been in the vanguard of efforts to devise public and private sector solutions to the problem of medical care financing and access.

The Unmet Need for Medical Care

As noted, if being underinsured is defined as having a 1% chance of having out-of-pocket medical expenses exceeding 10% of family income, then about 13% of Americans with insurance are inadequately insured.[40] By this standard, the 15 to 17% of Americans who are uninsured are also inadequately insured.* Therefore, 28 to 30% of Americans, from 58.8 to 63.0 million people, risk a serious financial burden. Two-thirds of the uninsured and one-half of the underinsured have incomes under 200% of the poverty level.[40,46] The threat of medical costs for these 34 million inadequately insured people creates not only financial stress but very likely a hurdle to access into the medical care system.

Do the approximately 60 million Americans who are inadequately insured actually face barriers to medical care? As noted above, in 1986, 39 million people reported difficulty in obtaining needed care and 1 million were unable to get care at all because of its cost.[3] This figure may, of course, overstate need, because people may seek unnecessary care, or it may understate it, because some are unaware of their need. The poor, minorities, and the uninsured use fewer physician services, despite their worse health status. Use, however, does not accurately measure need, because utilization may be insufficient or excessive. A more objective measure, defined by health professionals, is use adjusted for defined need[44] or use by subpopulations, such as children, pregnant women, or the chronically ill, for whom medical care is effective in both health and economic terms. Millions of people with a specific need for physician contact, such as young children, pregnant women, and people with high blood pressure, do not receive the routine medical surveillance that can improve their health and save long-term costs to the medical care system.[13] It is not possible with available data, however, to quantify the total extent of unmet need for medical care in the United States.

As is discussed in the next chapter, many of the uninsured poor are served by a variety of public programs and the charity care of hospitals and individual practitioners; others make difficult

---

*In 1977 dollars, all families with incomes under $60,000 would have a 1% chance of having out-of-pocket medical costs over 10% of income ($6,000).[40] Because most of the uninsured had incomes under $60,000, almost all the uninsured appear to have been underinsured.

choices, sacrificing basic needs to pay for medical care for their families. Still others postpone or delay care until their conditions become urgent or emergent, when they know that the local hospital emergency room is unlikely to refuse to treat them.

The great difficulty for policy makers in defining and describing the problem of access to medical care is estimating accurately the size of the population at risk. The temptation to state the problem in its broadest terms to focus needed public attention must be tempered with the concern that many state and national legislators pale at the apparent enormity of the problem. On the other hand, easing their worries by underestimating the population requiring care means risking an inadequate budget or insufficient public commitment and a program that cannot deliver on its promise of service to intended beneficiaries, a problem that has plagued Medicaid since its enactment. For these reasons, as well as the limitations on current public agency budgets, state and local governments addressing the issue recently have begun to divide the population into more manageable segments, such as mothers and children, the medically uninsurable, the unemployed, the elderly poor, or the working uninsured, so that they can tailor policy solutions to smaller groups. These new, targeted initiatives are examined in Chapter 3. The next chapter focuses on current public and private sources of funding for medical care for the poor and uninsured.

2

Who Finances Medical Care for the Poor, Uninsured, and Underinsured?

Traditional sources of medical care for people without insurance are declining. The public and private sectors have long financed and provided care to uninsured people, especially the poor, through a variety of programs. Although these commitments continue, their scope is decreasing because of the continuing high rate of increase in medical care expenditures, tight public budgets, and pressures on hospitals to lower prices in the newly competitive medical care marketplace. Conflicting demands placed on the public and private sectors have generated the public policy dilemma in financing indigent care, a quandary that grows as the number of uninsured people increases and as national medical care expenditures increase. An understanding of existing public and private sources of funding for indigent care is a necessary foundation for exploring solutions to this policy problem.

Public Sector Programs for the Poor and Uninsured

State and local governments have historically accepted responsibility for the poor under their constitutional jurisdiction to legislate for the public health and welfare. All states have authority to provide health care for the needy, and virtually all impose an obligation to do so on some level of government: state, county, or municipality. The programs established to perform this public duty remain the last resort by which millions of uninsured poor people can obtain medical care. But the Medicaid program, enacted 20 years ago to require federal and state governments to share financing of indigent care, must be included in any description of programs for the uninsured for several reasons: First, it is the primary source of funds for medical care to the poor; second, it is perceived as having contributed to increases in per capita medical care expenditures and inflation in medical care prices; third, it appears to have improved the health of its beneficiaries; and, finally, Medicaid expansion is the first step many states have taken to reduce the size of their uninsured populations, and it could form the basis for a national health program for the uninsured.

Medicaid

History of Medicaid.   Medicaid was enacted as Title XIX of the 1965 Social Security Act Amendments to complement Medicare, Title XVIII. Although in 1987 Medicaid was a $49.5 billion program serving 24 million beneficiaries, when enacted it was a "sleeper" that was somewhat hastily appended to the legislation for health insurance for the aged, which had been debated extensively for 4 years.[52] The crux of that debate was whether a health insurance program for the elderly should be centrally financed and administered through the Social Security program or whether it should be a more limited state and federal system of subsidizing private insurance, the alternative favored by organized medicine, the insurance industry, and the states.

In 1965 a three-part program was designed to defuse opposition to financing health care for the elderly: Hospital Insurance for the Aged (Medicare Part A, financed by Social Security payroll taxes), Supplementary Medical Insurance for the Aged (Medicare Part B, to pay for physician care, financed by subscriber premiums plus federal general revenues), and Medicaid (to pay for health care for the low-income elderly and other poor people, financed jointly by state and federal revenues but structured and administered by states). Medicaid was conceived as a program to distribute more equitably the costs of charity care, previously borne by providers and state and local governments. It is not clear that its drafters foresaw the extent to which Medicaid would support the elderly or fill the many gaps in Medicare, but hindsight reveals the symbiosis of the two programs. Although the public views Medicaid as a medical program for welfare mothers and children, its budget primarily funds services for the elderly and disabled, including nursing home care, which is not covered by Medicare.

Although Medicaid is now thought of as a medical program, it was originally structured as an extension of the existing welfare programs of income grants for families with dependent children and for aged, blind, and disabled adults. These welfare programs had paid for some medical care, first as part of the individual income supports and beginning in 1950 as "vendor payments" directly to medical care providers. The model for Medicaid was the Kerr-Mills program of Health Care for the Aged enacted by Congress in 1960.[53] Kerr-Mills was the first medical financing program that set minimum requirements for eligibility and services that states must offer the elderly poor to share in federal financing. The federal funding formula was designed to favor low-income states. The program recognized that many of the elderly poor who do not receive welfare can afford basic subsistence but not the cost of medical care, and it explicitly allowed for these "medically (not financially) needy" elderly to be eligible for assistance. The medically needy included not just people with incomes slightly above welfare levels, but also people with middle incomes who are faced with catastrophic illness. Kerr-Mills introduced the concept of "spending down" into medical assistance eligibility—that is, if net income after deducting health care expenses was below the eligibility standard for the medically needy, then a person became eligible for public funding of additional medical costs. This sliding-deductible feature of Kerr-Mills theoretically provided a sort of catastrophic insurance plan for even moderate-income elderly people.

Structure of Medicaid. Kerr-Mills was not viewed as very successful because few states adopted it, but its structure formed the foundation for Medicaid, which was described in 1965 as merely an extension of Kerr-Mills to additional groups of welfare recipients: the disabled and blind (now recipients of Supplemental Security Income, SSI) and welfare families (Aid to Families with Dependent Children, AFDC) where one parent was absent, disabled, or, in some states, unemployed. These welfare groups constitute Medicaid's "categorically needy" population. No public benefits program is technically "insurance" because subscribers do not share actuarial risk. But like Medicare, Medicaid was designed to resemble private health insurance plans with inpatient and outpatient benefits and cost-based payments for providers. As originally enacted, Medicaid required as a condition of receiving federal funds that a state provide to at least all its welfare recipient groups (categorically needy) a basic set of health services: inpatient and outpatient hospital care, physician services, laboratory and x-ray services, and skilled nursing home services. Additional mandatory services (rural clinic services, home health care, medical screening for children, and family planning services) were added in subsequent amendments to the law. States were allowed to cover virtually any other type of health care they might wish, such as prescription drugs, intermediate nursing home care, optometry, dental care, mental health care, medical equipment, and prosthetic devices.

States also were given broad discretion to add other groups of beneficiaries—for instance, people eligible for welfare but not receiving it for various reasons, children over 18 in school, and children in two-parent intact (non-AFDC) families. An additional group of beneficiaries that states could add were the Kerr-Mills-type medically needy people who meet the categorical requirements (age, blindness, disability, or a family with dependent children) but who have incomes and assets slightly above welfare levels and who are therefore deemed able to afford basic living costs but not medical care. If a state added such a group, it was also required to permit people to "spend down" into eligibility by deducting medical costs from income. This feature provides some protection from medical catastrophes for people just above the Medicaid income eligibility level and is particularly useful for nursing home residents. But because income eligibility levels are by law connected to state welfare payment levels and therefore very low, and because beneficiaries may possess only a limited amount of property, the "spend down" does not provide the medically needy with the broad catastrophic protection that may have been originally intended.

Financing of Medicaid. To encourage state participation, Congress provided for open-ended federal financial matching of from 50% to 83% of a state's costs. Poorer states, such as those in the South, receive a higher federal share than do richer states, according to a formula based on the difference between a state's per capita income and the national average. The federal government splits costs of program administration 50–50 with the states. But to encourage certain activities, such as the development of computerized claims processing, fraud control units, provision of family planning services, and utilization review by peer review groups, Congress provided for a higher federal matching rate for some services. For example, for information systems, fraud control, and family planning, the federal match is 90%; for peer review, it is 75%.

State Medicaid Programs. By 1970, all states but Arizona had adopted Medicaid programs, varying widely in benefits, eligibility requirements, budget, and administration.* About two-thirds of the states cover the medically needy, and most cover many optional services, such as prescription drugs, eyeglasses, dental care, and nursing home care for the mentally retarded. Because Medicaid expenditures exceeded early estimates and were held responsible for growth in national medical care expenditures, Congress enacted limits on medically needy eligibility levels, permitted states to reduce programs, provided controls on benefits, and allowed states to require some Medicaid recipients to pay part of the costs of their care. Given broader discretion to reduce benefits and services, during the 1970s many states cut their programs and imposed limits on covered services, such as the number of hospital days or physician visits per beneficiary. Although some optionally covered groups were also eliminated during this decade, the most severe cuts in Medicaid eligibility came in 1980, when Congress cut about 440,000 working welfare mothers from AFDC welfare eligibility, causing at least 1.2 million mothers and children to lose Medicaid eligibility.[55]

Recent Changes in Medicaid. Considering the tide of program cuts, it was surprising to see Congress expand eligibility during the 1980s. For the first time, in 1981, states could add a limited "medically needy" program covering only pregnant women and children

---

*Arizona adopted an experimental medical assistance program in 1982. It requires all beneficiaries to be enrolled in organized health care provider systems. It covers no long-term care, although the state is now considering adding such services.[54]

in AFDC (generally single-parent) households, rather than being required to add all AFDC households plus the aged, blind, and disabled. This change was designed to be a program limitation, because it gave states greater flexibility to eliminate the "comparability" of treatment of different welfare groups, but it has actually helped states expand Medicaid coverage, because they can add a group for whom health care is both inexpensive and cost-effective without also adding the most costly medically needy groups, the aged and disabled.

As a result of Social Security Act amendments in 1984 (PL 96–369), 1985 (PL 99–272), 1986 (PL 99–509), 1987 (PL 100–203), and 1988 (PL 100–360), states are now required to cover children from birth to 6 years of age, pregnant women in two-parent families with incomes below AFDC standards, and by 1990 pregnant women and children aged 0–1 with incomes up to the poverty level. States are also allowed to cover at their option pregnant women, children under age 8 (phased in through 1991), the elderly, and the disabled, all of whom may be members of families with incomes as high as the federal poverty line, and children under age 1 and pregnant women with incomes up to 185% of the poverty line. Because income eligibility levels for most state Medicaid programs are less than half of the federal poverty level,[56] this new option allows many more poor people to be covered. These changes, especially those in PL 99–509 and PL 100–203, have gradually detached Medicaid from its historic link to welfare. Welfare reform bills in the 100th Congress would also mandate AFDC and Medicaid coverage of two-parent families with unemployed parents and would extend Medicaid eligibility for employed workers leaving welfare.

Another important change to the Medicaid law was the 1981 mandate (reinforced in 1987 by PL 100–203) that states provide extra reimbursement to hospitals providing a disproportionate share of care to the poor; fewer than half the states have explicitly done so, however.[57]

Medicaid's Impact on Health Status. It is well recognized that Medicaid has increased access to inpatient and ambulatory services for 24 million poor people. For instance, before 1965 the poor had fewer physician visits than the non-poor, but shortly after Medicaid's enactment the per capita hospital stays and physician visits of the poor exceeded those of higher income groups (Figure

1.1). If the lower health status of the poor is considered, per capita physician visits were approximately equal.[19,42] Recent evidence suggests, however, that the poor's use of medical care may have declined relative to that of higher income groups.[13]

It is reasonable to conclude that the health status of the poor who are eligible for Medicaid has improved since its enactment. The national decline in infant mortality accelerated sharply in 1965 although at a lower rate for blacks than whites.[25] In 1970, the overall U.S. age-adjusted death rate also began a precipitous decline,[25] attributable to technological improvements in medical care as well as increased access. Although environmental and social factors and other initiatives of the War on Poverty programs of the mid-1960s have also contributed to lower death rates, it is more than coincidental that health status improvements were manifest in the late 1960s as states adopted Medicaid programs. As more pregnant women and children become covered by the program, it will be important to see whether low birth weight and infant mortality and morbidity improve concomitantly.

Medicaid's Problems. Despite the obvious benefits of Medicaid, it suffers from several serious limitations. First is its continued connection to the welfare income-support programs. Although states may now cover pregnant women, young children, the elderly, and the disabled in nonwelfare families with incomes as high as or higher than the poverty level, Medicaid coverage remains primarily based on welfare eligibility categories; thus, most single adults who are not elderly or totally disabled, most childless couples, most nonpregnant parents in two-parent families, and many older children are not eligible to participate. Another problem with Medicaid's welfare connection, especially in states without programs for the medically needy, is the transient nature of the coverage. Eligibility status frequently changes as people move in and out of employment or change income levels slightly.

Furthermore, tying general Medicaid income eligibility to welfare levels, which are well below the poverty level in most states and have not kept pace with inflation, assures that the program will cover only a fraction of the poor. Medicaid was estimated to cover fewer than half of the population below the poverty level in 1984, down from a high of 65% in 1976[58] (Figure 2.1). In fact, while the number of people in poverty was increasing from 1978 to 1983, the

Fig. 2.1—Medicaid recipients as a percentage of the population with incomes at or below 125% of the poverty level, 1969–85. (In 1983 the poverty level for a family of four was $10,178 and median income was $33,212.)

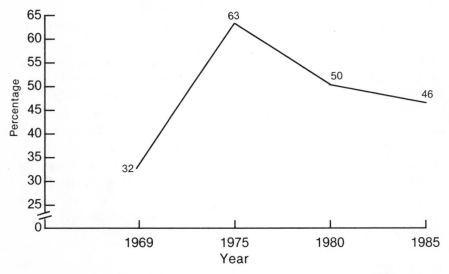

Source: U.S. Senate Special Committee on Aging, 99th Congress, 1st Session. Americans at risk: The case of the medically uninsured; 1985.

number of people receiving Medicaid remained nearly constant (Figure 2.2).

An additional structural problem with Medicaid is the discretion given to states to design programs within general federal guidelines. The ability to choose among various eligibility standards, covered services, and administrative approaches makes Medicaid not one but 50 different programs.[59] Despite the more generous federal financing of the poorer Southern states, they have the most limited programs in terms of benefits and eligibility. Thus, only 24% of people under the federal poverty level are covered in Alabama, compared with 83% in California.[60] It must be acknowledged that the state discretion built into Medicaid has allowed some states to meet local needs by creative and innovative experimentation with new forms of medical care delivery, such as the case management program in Michigan. Greater uniformity in eligibility and benefits could be encouraged, however, to eliminate interstate inequities.

Fig. 2.2—Number of Medicaid recipients and people below the poverty level in the United States, 1972–84. The ratio of Medicaid recipients to persons below the poverty level is given in parentheses above each year.

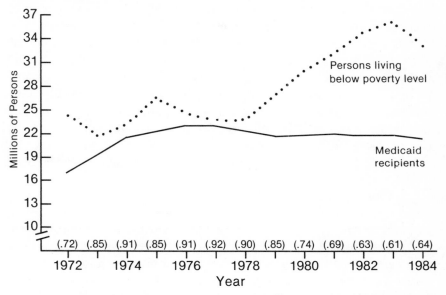

Source: Gornick M, Greenberg J, Eggers P, Dobson A. Twenty years of Medicaid and Medicare: Covered populations, use of benefits, and program expenditures. Health Care Financing Review 1985;(Suppl):34.

Another difficulty with Medicaid has been its reliance on voluntary medical care providers. In adopting Medicare and Medicaid, Congress prohibited any government "interference" in the practice of medicine, an admonition that seems largely lost today with the active oversight of medical care costs and use under these programs. Despite these controls, however, providers (other than hospitals that have received Hill-Burton construction funds) can choose not to accept Medicare or Medicaid patients. Although the existence of substantial government funding has encouraged the growth of whole industries, such as nursing homes, the program's increasing administrative complexities (payment levels that fail to keep pace with inflation, reimbursement delays, and constant changes) have discouraged many providers from participating. This has been a particular problem for physicians. It is estimated that fewer than half of practicing physicians take Medicaid patients in many states,[61] and participation varies widely by specialty.[62] Also, many nursing homes limit their Medicaid admissions.

The distribution of payments among Medicaid beneficiaries is also a source of complaints. Just over one-quarter of the recipients (the aged, blind, and disabled) use three-quarters of the budget, whereas families and children constitute the largest category of recipients but receive disproportionately fewer program dollars.[63] This maldistribution is largely due to the costs of nursing home care for the elderly and the developmentally disabled (mentally retarded), who account for more than 40% of the national Medicaid budget.[61] The group receiving the most funding is the elderly, who in 1984 received 36.5% of national Medicaid budget expenditures in payments for nursing home care, Medicare's premiums and cost sharing, and services not covered by Medicare, such as prescription drugs and eyeglasses.[61]

A final problem with the Medicaid program has been the public's perception that it, along with Medicare, is responsible for continued increases in per capita as well as overall medical care expenditures. Both Medicaid and Medicare are entitlement programs—that is, they pay for certain benefits for anyone meeting defined eligibility criteria. Unlike categorical programs that need cover eligibles only to the extent of a fixed budget, Medicaid and Medicare must cover costs of all enrollees, even if this requires supplemental appropriations or cutting benefits or costs.

Increased demand for medical care was facilitated by the availability of health insurance and cost-based reimbursement for institutions in the first 15 years of Medicaid and Medicare, and this increased demand certainly contributed to the growth of medical care expenditures. However, government responses, such as review of the appropriateness of hospital admissions, prospective payment, case management, and risk-sharing contracts, brought rates of expenditure increases for Medicaid below those for general medical care from 1981 to 1985.[48] Spending increases in subsequent years have been close to 11%, partially resulting from increased eligibility under the recent congressional expansions. State programs have also become models for private sector health care purchasers struggling with medical care cost containment. Other contributors to growing medical care spending, such as increased volume and intensity of care, are endemic in the U.S. health care system and cannot so easily be traced to the public payment programs. But the image of Medicaid as a "budget buster" is pervasive among legislators. The increasingly large share of state budgets devoted to Medicaid, often due to long-term care payments, leaves Medicaid politically vulnerable to reduction pressures.

Medicaid's limitations in no way undermine the importance of the program as a source of funding for medical care for millions of poor Americans. In fact, the program's strengths, including its innovations in health care delivery systems and cost containment, could be used to fashion a more equitable and far-reaching program of medical care for the nation's poor, as discussed in Chapter 4.

Medicare

Medicare was envisioned as a medical care program for all the elderly, not just those who are poor. (Medicaid was expressly adopted to meet the needs of the elderly who are unable to afford the costs unpaid by Medicare.) Nevertheless, it offers financial protection for elderly people, many of whom could not afford to purchase health care. About a quarter of all Medicare beneficiaries are below the federal poverty level.[38] Because of private pensions and Social Security payments that keep pace with inflation, the overall economic status of the elderly has improved dramatically in recent years. But although a smaller proportion of elderly people than children, for instance, fall below the federal poverty line, a third of them have incomes near the poverty level and would be considered unable to afford medical care if Medicare and Medicaid did not pay for it.[64] Furthermore, many of the near-poor elderly are ineligible for Medicaid and are financially stressed by the medical care costs unpaid by Medicare, such as costs of drugs, copayments, deductibles, and Part B premiums, all of which have increased steadily.[38]

Medicare is administered by the federal government, which contracts with private insurers to process claims. Part A covers hospital care, limited nursing home benefits, and home health care for people who are eligible for Social Security payments and are at least 65 years old or have been permanently disabled for at least 2 years. (The few people not automatically eligible for Social Security can subscribe to Part A by paying a monthly premium, $250 in 1987.) Part B covers physician services, medical equipment, prosthetic devices, and additional home health care for elderly or disabled people who pay a monthly premium ($18 in 1987), regardless of Social Security eligibility.

The $78-billion program (serving 33 million beneficiaries in 1987) has been plagued with financial problems because expenditures have increased faster than revenues, and several steps have been taken to control utilization and costs, including limiting fees to various providers, such as physicians; mandating utilization reviews; and paying hospitals prospectively. Because the federal government is the largest single purchaser of hospital services through Medicare, it has enormous leverage over the way hospital care is financed and delivered. The government's exercise of that influence, for instance by its prospective payment (diagnosis related group, DRG) system, is bound to change health care delivery dramatically in the future.

The Medicare program is an indispensable source of medical care payment for its millions of beneficiaries, although it covers less than half of the medical care costs of elderly people. Medicare has recently survived threats to the financial integrity of its trust funds. Debates over the program are inconsistent. In 1985 they focused on alternative financing arrangements, such as increased income-based cost sharing by beneficiaries; in 1987 they involved improving coverage to protect beneficiaries from catastrophic costs, financing these changes by increasing monthly premiums and income tax surcharges for wealthier Medicare beneficiaries.

Federal Categorical Programs

The federal government funds many programs that provide medical services to the poor in addition to Medicare and Medicaid, hospital and nursing home care for veterans, and health insurance for federal employees, military personnel, and their dependents. These programs target special populations, such as mothers and children, Indians, migrants, and substance abusers, and are generally administered by state or local public health agencies. In 1987 they cost more than $2.5 billion. Included in this figure is $400 million that supports about half the operating budgets of 550 rural and urban community health centers that serve more than 5 million persons. The 125 migrant health centers serve 2.7 million migrant and seasonal farm workers at a cost of $45.4 million. The maternal and child health block grant of $478 million provides prenatal and well child care to millions of poor mothers and children. The Indian Health Service is funded at almost $1 billion to serve Native Americans living on and off reservations. About $550 million of the federal budget funds alcohol and drug abuse prevention and treatment programs.

All of these programs are important sources of specific services for their intended populations, but because of budget limits they meet only some of the need. Although current federal budgets for these programs appear stable, in 1982, 250 community health centers were closed by funding cuts. These federal programs are constantly threatened by funding reductions or termination.

State and Local Indigent Medical Care Programs

Long before the federal government assumed a role in welfare programs for the poor, state and local governments had undertaken these responsibilities. States are authorized to provide for the health and welfare of their populations through the "police powers" reserved to them under the Tenth Amendment to the U.S. Constitution. In all states, statutes authorize various levels of government to provide some medical care for their residents. In all but three states, either state or local governments are statutorily or constitutionally obligated to provide at least some health services to some indigent populations (Table 2.1). These requirements derive from Elizabethan "poor laws," which were widely adopted by states in the 19th century. They are legal obligations that have been enforced increasingly by patients as well as hospitals and physicians seeking payment for their charity care.[65] During fiscal year 1982, state and local programs were estimated to have cost $15 billion (in addition to the states' $16 billion share of Medicaid costs that year).[66]

Although statutory duties are important to determine the government agency ultimately responsible for indigent medical care, actual operating programs in many states do not always comply with the statutes (Table 2.1). For instance, 24 states have sole or partial legal responsibility for indigent care, but 34 states actually operate state or state/local programs. Counties in Kansas are liable for indigent care under the state constitution, but the state currently finances and administers a statewide program for the poor. In contrast, the programs in some states with legal obligations are so limited that many counties, especially those operating hospitals and clinics, provide more basic medical care to their residents than the state requires. Furthermore, some states operate programs with no express statutory authority, legislating medical care for the poor through state budget acts. For instance, for many years Colorado operated a $30-million indigent care program with no authority other than the annual budget bill.

Recent surveys provide extensive data about state medical care programs for the poor and uninsured.[67] Although the 50 states' indigent care activities vary much more than their Medicaid programs, there are a handful of basic approaches. Many of the 3,000 counties in the United States also provide health care for the poor, but very little is known about the operation or costs of their programs. County programs generally follow the same models as those at the state level, but there are no data on the prevalence of the various approaches. Thirty-four states operate 41 different state programs, some in conjunction with counties or municipalities.[67] In these states, programs often vary greatly from county to county. State and local indigent care programs can be characterized by the levels of government legally responsible for operating financing, and administering them, as well as by their basic structural differences.

Indigent Care Program Approaches

From a structural viewpoint, state and local medical care programs for the poor can be distinguished by their focus on either individual patients or institutions (Table 2.1). Those that target individuals, providing dollars to follow the patient rather than to support institutions, are often based on entitlement models, such as Medicaid.

Programs Targeting Individuals. Several states have adopted state-financed Medicaid-type programs for the populations not covered by Medicaid: single adults, childless couples, and intact families (Table 2.1). Services covered under these state-only programs are usually similar to Medicaid services, but income eligibility levels may be lower. The most popular Medicaid-type programs are a medical component to general relief (GR) or general assistance (GA) programs. GR and GA programs provide income support for

(Text continues on page 44.)

Table 2.1—Characteristics of State and Local Programs of Health Care for the Poor and Uninsured

State	Level of Government Responsible — Legal Obligation[a]	Administration[b]	Financing	Type of Program — Individual	Institution	Mandatory Hospital Rate Setting	Insurance Risk Pool[b]	Hospital Emergency Care Mandate[a]	Insurance Continuation[b]	Insurance Conversion[b]
Alabama	C[d]	C	C							
Alaska[e]	S	S	S	X						
Arizona	C	C, S	C, S						X	X
Arkansas	C[f], S	S	C, S		X				X	X
California	C	C	C, S							X
Colorado	S[g]	S	C[g], S		X					X
Connecticut	T, S[h]	T, S	T, S	X		X			X	X
Delaware	S	C	C				X		X	X
DC	Dist	Dist	Dist							
Florida	C[i]	C	C, S				X		X	X
Georgia	C[j], S	C	C							X
Hawaii[j]	S	S	S	X						
Idaho	C	C	C							
Illinois	C, S	C, S	C, S	X			X	X		X
Indiana	T, C	S	C, S		X		X			
Iowa	C	C, S	C, S	X			X		X	X
Kansas	C[k], S	S	S	X					X	X
Kentucky	None	S	S		X			X	X	X
Louisiana	Parrish	P, S	P, S[l]		X			X	X	X
Maine[m]	T, S	T, S	T, S	X		X	X		X	X
Maryland	S	C, S	S	X		X		X	X	X
Massachusetts	S	S	S	X		X		X	X	X
Michigan	C	C, S	C, S	X					X	X
Minnesota[d]	T, C	C, S	T, C, S	X			X		X	X

Table 2.1—Continued

State	Level of Government Responsible			Type of Program		Mandatory Hospital Rate Setting	Insurance Risk Pool[b]	Hospital Emergency Care Mandate[a]	Insurance Continuation[b]	Insurance Conversion[b]
	Legal Obligation[a]	Admin-istration[b]	Financing	Individual	Institution					
Mississippi	C[d], S	S	None (abandoned in favor of Medicaid)		X					
Missouri	C	S	S	X				X	X	X
Montana	C	C, S	C, S	X			X		X	X
Nebraska	C, S	C	C				X		X	
Nevada	C	C	C							X
New Hampshire[m]	T, C	T, C	T, C	X					X	X
New Jersey	T, S	T, S	T, S			X		X		
New Mexico	C, S[n]	C	C, S[n]		X				X	X
New York	C	C, S	C, S	X		X		X	X	X
North Carolina	None[g]	C	C[g]							
North Dakota	C	C	C, S				X			
Ohio	C	C, S	C, S	X					X	X
Oklahoma	C	C, S	C, S		X				X	X
Oregon	S	S	S	X				X	X	X
Pennsylvania	C	S	S	X				X		X
Rhode Island[m]	T, S	T, C, S	T, C, S	X			X	X	X	X
South Carolina	S	S	S		X				X	X
South Dakota	C, S	C, S	C, S							X
Tennessee	None	–	None				X	X	X	
Texas	C	C	C, S					X		
Utah	C	S	C, S					X		X
Vermont	S	S	S	X						

State							
Virginia	C, S	C, S	C, S		X		X	X
Washington	S[g]	S	S		X		X	X
West Virginia	S	—	None		X		X	X
Wisconsin	T, C	T	T, C, S	X		X	X	X
Wyoming	S[g]	S	S[g]	X		X	X	X

Key—S = State; C = County; T = Town/Municipality.

[a] Source: Butler P. Legal obligations of state and local governments for indigent health care. In: Curtis R, ed. Access to care for the medically indigent: a resource document for state and local officials. Washington, DC: Academy for State and Local Government, 1985.

[b] Source: Desonia R, King K. State programs of assistance for the medically indigent. Washington, DC: Intergovernmental Health Policy Project, George Washington University, 1985.

[c] Source: Dowell MA. Indigent access to hospital emergency room services. Clearinghouse Rev 1984;5:483–499.

[d] Statute expressly requires counties to pay for out-of-county hospital care but does not mention in-county care.

[e] State has catastrophic illness program that is not currently funded.

[f] Counties are liable to state university medical center hospital for care of counties' indigent residents.

[g] If county operates a hospital, it must treat indigents free.

[h] State is responsible for people without a town of residence.

[i] County liable to pay hospital for emergency care of pregnant women in labor.

[j] State law requires private employers to insure employees.

[k] Counties are liable under state constitution, although state operates an indigent health care program.

[l] Indigents are eligible for free care at state indigent care hospitals.

[m] State operates a catastrophic illness expense program.

[n] State program limited to coverage of aged, blind, or disabled people who are severely ill.

the poor who are eligible for nonfederal welfare, but many GA and GR programs have lower income levels than those under AFDC or SSI and some have requirements that recipients be disabled or unemployable.[68] A dozen states provide medical assistance, often similar to the coverage of their Medicaid programs but in some cases limited to hospital or ambulatory care, to recipients of GA or GR. Several other state indigent care programs use a Medicaid model unconnected to GA or GR.

Other public medical care programs targeting poor people include those providing maternal and child health care (often partially federally funded) or care to senior citizens. Still other state programs focus on specific diseases (eg, cancer and hemophilia) or services (eg, eyeglasses, prescription drugs, and dentures).

States also assist uninsured people through insurance regulation by creating risk pools for uninsurables or requiring continuation or conversion of group health insurance[69] (Table 2.1). These approaches are discussed further in Chapter 3.

Of four states with statutory catastrophic insurance programs that pay for very costly illness of their residents, only those in New Hampshire and Rhode Island are currently funded. Because of the costliness of these programs and concerns about budget unpredictability, no states have enacted general catastrophic programs in the past 10 years,[69] although in 1988 New Jersey adopted a program to cover children's catastrophic medical costs.

Programs Targeting Providers. Rather than structuring medical care programs to serve the poor through a public "insurance" approach, some state and local governments have designed them around institutions, primarily hospitals. The most common institutionally based indigent care model is the public hospital or clinic, a traditional source of medical care for the poor. In 1982 local governments spent $9.5 billion for such public institutions.[70] This model is sometimes also used by states operating public medical schools and university hospitals. A more prevalent state-level approach, however, is to target payments to private hospitals through grants or payment programs designed to defray some of the costs of hospital charity care. Although these programs obviously benefit uninsured patients, they are often politically supported as ways of maintaining public institutions, providing teaching material, or helping private hospitals that provide charity care to compete with less generous counterparts by leveling the competitive playing field among hospitals.

A regulatory approach to assist institutions is all-payer rate setting. Nine states regulate hospital charges to government and private payers (Table 2.1). The rates established for each institution include payment for the costs of charity and bad debt; in other words, these programs institutionalize cost shifting and spread it among all payers.* Rate setting does not discourage providers from rendering charity care or encourage patient dumping to other institutions because the care will be reimbursed. But these systems tend to sanction existing charity care patterns and may encourage treatment of the poor in relatively costly settings (inpatient or emergency rooms). In 1986 and 1987 Massachusetts and New Jersey changed the charity care features of their rate-setting programs to create pools that redistribute funds to hospitals with the highest indigent care loads and to more outpatient services.[71]

Another regulatory approach is to mandate that hospitals provide charity care. About half the states now prohibit hospitals from turning away emergency cases,[72] a requirement similar to Medicare's limitations on transfer enacted by Congress in 1986 (PL 99-272). As of 1987 no state required a minimum charity care contribution as a condition of a hospital's operating license, although the Texas legislature tried, without success, to impose such an obligation in 1984, and in 1987 Maine's hospital rate-setting commission developed regulations to impose such a requirement. (New York requires home health agencies to provide a specified amount of free care.[73]) A few states require a showing of charity care for hospital capital expansions through certificate of need review. Many states allow charitable institutions to be exempt from state income and property taxes, and a few have interpreted this exemption to apply to medical care providers only if they provide some charity care. The Utah Supreme Court, for instance, mandated inquiry into each hospital's charity care policies, its use of capital for construction compared to charity care, and the extent of actual discounts to the poor.[74] A Vermont superior court, however, has held that free care is not a prerequisite to property tax exemption.[75]

---

*Medicare participates in rate setting under waivers of federal law only in Maryland and New Jersey.

Demands on Public Programs

It is impossible to estimate how many poor and uninsured people are served by such state and local government programs, but their number is substantial. In many parts of the country, these government agencies have experienced increasing demands for other public services and declining revenues and are especially stressed by continued increases in per capita medical care expenditures. Although some states and localities have rebounded from the recession earlier in this decade, others, notably those with economies based on oil, face hard times in the late 1980s and are wary of patients' and private providers' expectations that state and local government will fulfill legal or moral duties as a last-resort source of funding for indigent care. Local public hospitals have been particularly hard hit; many have closed or been sold or leased to private management firms, which retain legal responsibility for indigent care but are primarily concerned about a healthy bottom line.[76] Most public hospitals have struggled to become more price competitive as their tax subsidies have failed to keep pace with increasing demand and their need to retain privately insured patients has become more obvious. Public facilities are facing pressures similar to their counterparts in the private sector.

Private Sector Financing of Indigent Care

The preponderance of American medical care is financed through the private sector; about three-quarters of the population under age 65 is privately insured. Two-thirds of this coverage comes through the workplace and is funded largely by employers. Most other insurance is privately purchased, often to supplement Medicare and other public programs. As noted in Chapter 1, private sector coverage appears to be declining (Table 1.2). In addition to firms that no longer offer insurance and an increasing number of service firms, which have never offered it, many businesses have increased cost sharing by enrollees and have adopted coverage limits. Although medical care cost containment is appropriate, it should not be an excuse to erode the important protection that employer-sponsored health insurance represents to the American public.

Even for the uninsured, the private sector plays an important role in financing care. Private sector medical care providers have a tradition of charity and community service similar to that of public providers. In fact, the modern hospital developed from the parallel history of public institutions for the poor, the mentally ill, and patients with infectious diseases and from the religious-affiliated private, nonprofit hospitals for the poor.[77]

Philanthropy

As a percentage of all personal U.S. health care expenditures, philanthropy represents a small share: 1.2% or about $3.4 billion in 1982, a slight decline from 1.4% in 1976.[66] The American Hospital Association (AHA) estimated that in 1984, philanthropy accounted for 4% of average capital financing of U.S. hospitals.* It is generally acknowledged that almost all gifts to hospitals are dedicated for capital projects—donors prefer tangible evidence of their contributions—rather than for operating expenses for the poor or other non-self-supporting activities. Therefore, total philanthropic contribution to hospitals is not likely to exceed 4 to 5% of hospital costs. A 1983 survey of Colorado hospitals showed that less than 3% of their charitable donations were used for uncompensated care.[78] Philanthropy paid for only 4% of indigent care in California hospitals.[79] Philanthropic support of hospitals declined with the advent of public and private third-party payment.[80]

Many local charities, such as United Way agencies and low-income patient clinics, benefit from private gifts to support their operating costs of medical care for the poor. Private philanthropy could provide a greater source of charity care than it has in the past if tax laws, which provide varying incentives for individuals and businesses to make charitable contributions, were more consistently applied toward a policy of encouraging greater private philanthropy for the uninsured poor.

Charity Care by Physicians and Other Practitioners

Professional ethics are the foundation of a tradition of charity care among physicians, but neither the extent, the type, nor the settings of these voluntary services is well documented. A survey by the American Medical Association (AMA) revealed that three-quarters of American physicians provided some free or discounted

---

*Personal communication, research staff, American Hospital Association, Chicago.

health care to patients in 1982.[81] Identical findings resulted from a survey of Colorado physicians the same year.[78] Little is known about the value that this charity represents.* Organized medicine developed many special programs to assist the recently unemployed and uninsured during the recession in the early 1980s, and it is unclear whether the survey figures are typical of times when such publicized efforts are not under way. Certainly, in the many states where Medicaid fees have failed to keep pace with inflation, physicians participating in Medicaid render a significant charity contribution.

Even less is known about the manner in which physicians finance charity care. Some physicians augment the staff of public or nonprofit health centers for free or at reduced charges, but the major proportion of physician charity is probably provided through individual patient contacts in the private physician's office, in some cases for existing patients fallen on hard times and in other cases for new patients accepted explicitly as charity cases. Whether physicians consciously raise charges to paying patients to compensate for nonpaying cases is not known. Although some charity care is undoubtedly undertaken as a community service, to the extent that physicians "target" income and patient volume,[50,83] it is likely that paying patients subsidize at least some of the costs of unpaid charity care.

It would be easier, however, for physicians rather than hospitals to absorb charity care costs without raising prices to other patients. That is, self-employed individuals or small partnerships have more flexibility than corporations, which must pay all employees' salaries, to choose to provide extra, unbillable care. This hypothesis is consistent with the AMA survey finding that self-employed physicians were more likely than physician employees to provide free care.[81] As the supply of physicians increases and their incomes decline or as they increasingly work for HMOs and other employers, physicians may be less willing to increase charity care or even to continue it at current levels.

---

*The AMA survey data showed that each respondent provided $16,000 in charity care during 1982, for a national total of $9 billion. One analyst feels that this total is "implausibly high" as a result of response bias.[82] Surveys in Colorado have shown that physicians do not have good records of the value of this care and must therefore provide rough estimates.

There are no data available on the charity care provided by other health care practitioners, although a large share of members of other long-standing professions, such as nursing and chiropractic, undoubtedly provide similar, unmeasured contributions.

Uncompensated Care by Hospitals

Today 58% of all U.S. hospitals are private, not-for-profit corporations with community boards of directors. Publicly owned hospitals constitute another 28%, and proprietary (for-profit) hospitals make up the remaining 14%. Because of their public or philanthropic genesis, most hospitals have long espoused a charitable mission of community service, many explicitly to care for the poor. These traditional commitments have been underscored by legal requirements. For instance, hospitals receiving Hill-Burton construction grants or loans were expressly mandated to provide free care (calculated as 3% of their operating costs) to low-income patients. In many states, hospitals with emergency rooms cannot turn away true emergency cases.[72] Recently enacted federal law (PL 99–272) prohibits hospitals participating in Medicare from transferring an emergency case without stabilizing the patient and arranging for transfer to another institution. This program suffers from lack of regulations, notice to beneficiaries, and federal enforcement.[10]

Considering these customs and mandates, it is not surprising that U.S. hospitals provide a large amount of free or discounted care. Although the term "uncompensated care" is widely used, as discussed in Chapter 1, its definition is subject to disagreement and controversy. Uncompensated care is often valued as unpaid charges, which vary among hospitals. It should be measured as a percentage of hospital costs. Furthermore, uncompensated care may include charity care, bad debt, negotiated discounts, and costs unpaid by Medicaid or Medicare. Thus, it may overstate the extent of costs for charity patients, because some bad debt may be collectible and because private sector discounts should not be included in a category for which public subsidies are sought. Finally, the $9.5-billion contribution of state and local governments for hospital care through non-Medicaid programs in 1982[70] should be considered when estimating the burden of uncompensated care on hospitals. A uniform national definition of unsponsored charity care would be very helpful to policy makers.

Mindful of the problem of defining uncompensated care, AHA recently estimated the costs of "unsponsored" care that hospitals bear—that is, the amount of charity care plus bad debt minus any state or local payments. AHA estimated that the cost of unsponsored care by all hospitals in 1984 was $5.7 billion, a 107% increase since 1980 and a real increase of 50%, considering inflation. Such care accounted for 3.6% of average hospital costs in 1980 and 4.6% in 1984.[60] It is unsponsored care that creates the need for hospitals to "cost shift"—that is, raise charges to paying patients to the extent possible to subsidize unpaid care. (Cost shifting is a misnomer, of course, because it is unclear which costs are actually charged to other payers. The cross-subsidy would be more appropriately called "revenue shifting.") Considering that charity cases constitute a small proportion of most hospitals' patient loads, these costs should be calculated as marginal costs. Hospitals do not account for them in this way, however. Regardless of how it is calculated, the subsidy for unsponsored care is an indirect tax on the few uninsured people who pay directly for hospital care and, more important, on the third-party insurers that have traditionally paid full costs for hospital services.

Were the burden of uncompensated or unsponsored care borne equally among most hospitals, it would not pose the policy dilemma it does because it could be seen as a private sector means of financing care for the uninsured. However, the distribution of charity care, uncompensated or unsponsored, varies widely among hospitals. For instance, half of U.S. hospitals devoted less than 6% of their costs to unsponsored care in 1984, but 5% of hospitals provided more than 10% of their costs as charity.[60] Public hospitals located in poor, inner-city areas and legally mandated to care for the poor bear the greatest share of uncompensated care,[81,84] but depending on the extent of their government revenues, public hospitals may have lower levels of unsponsored care than some private, nonprofit institutions.[60]

The charity service of proprietary hospitals is less well studied because of the small number of for-profit hospitals nationwide and their lack of response to national surveys. Some analysts have found no statistical differences in charity care between private, nonprofit, and for-profit hospitals.[82] Others have, however, noted considerable variation.[81] Some states with a large number of for-profit hospitals have learned, for instance, that although these hospitals do pay state and local taxes, they provide a lower share of uncompensated care than their nonprofit counterparts. As a percentage of gross revenue, in 1982 for-profit hospitals in Florida provided 0.2% charity care and 3.6% bad debt, compared with 1.8% and 4.8%, respectively, for nonprofit hospitals and 2.4% and 9.7%, respectively, for public hospitals.[85] Like other aggregate data, such broad statistics mask important differences in individual hospital commitments. Some for-profit hospitals serving as sole community providers give relatively large amounts of charity care, and some nonprofit institutions provide very little because of their favorable locations or public hospitals that bear the full burden.

Not only are some private and many public institutions providing a disproportionate share of charity care, many are financially stressed. Less than 9% of hospitals provided care for more than 40% of poor patients in 1980, and a third of these hospitals had deficits that year, which jeopardized their ability to meet community service needs.[47] Compared with financially stable hospitals serving similarly large proportions of the uninsured poor, these deficits derive from insufficient revenues from insured patients rather than from underuse or inefficiency. About 20% of hospitals with large poor patient populations adopted explicit limits on charity care in 1980.[47] (Characteristics of patients accounting for uncompensated care are described in Appendix B.)

To understand how uncompensated or unsponsored care meets the needs of the uninsured, it is necessary to examine how hospitals respond to increased demand. Is there a limit, for instance, to hospitals' ability to finance unsponsored care by raising charges to other patients? Analysis of data from the early 1980s suggests that in general hospitals are unable or unwilling to increase charity care to meet all increased need. The percentage of uninsured poor grew 20% from 1980 to 1982 (partly because of increased unemployment, increased numbers of people in poverty, and reductions in federal Medicaid eligibility), but hospital charity and bad debt increased only 3.8%.[70] Public hospitals responded most directly by providing more free care than private hospitals, but because of their limited public resources, they were unable to meet all the need. Private hospitals did increase their share of Medicaid patients slightly during this period, but because of limited Medicaid eligibility in some states, this action did not satisfy all needs.[70] Analysts have shown that at least during these years, hospitals did not significantly raise charges to private insurers to cover additional charity care.[86] Rather, they adopted explicit policies to ration free care by using budgetary quotas, requiring advance payment, and reducing services, such as outpatient care or social services programs.[70,86]

Hospital cost shifting has existed since the advent of third-party insurance and will undoubtedly continue. If Medicaid and Medicare fail to pay close to full costs for some patients and Blue Cross and other preferred insurers receive discounts, some paying patients will subsidize others. But cost shifting is being challenged by purchasers with enough bargaining power to demand more favorable treatment. The dilemma currently facing all medical care providers, especially hospitals, the target of many cost-containment initiatives, is how to compete on price in an increasingly tough medical care marketplace.

Medical care expenditure increases and the oversupply of hospital beds and physicians have spurred both government and private sector purchasers—especially employers and insurers—to become more prudent. They expect providers to discount prices and share financial risk. Hospitals have responded by cutting costs, laying off employees, and limiting charity care.[86] Reducing uncompensated care is easier for many hospitals than other cost-cutting measures. State and local health service budgets have failed to keep pace with medical care expenditure increases and the number of uninsured people has grown because of declining enrollment in private insurance and Medicaid, but hospitals have generally not expanded their free care commitment to meet this need. Hospitals, especially those under legal mandates, are likely to continue to shoulder some of the indigent care load. Their financial ability to do so will be limited if they respond to marketplace directives to reduce prices. The hospitals that do not respond are likely to lose insured patients, an important source of revenue to finance a portion of unsponsored care. Hospitals thus face a Hobson's choice in the current cost-conscious medical care market, and their uninsured patients will feel the effects of that choice in reduced access to care.

3

New Approaches to Financing and Delivering Care to the Poor, Uninsured, and Underinsured

As the number of uninsured poor people has grown, as public budgets have been restricted, and as hospitals have limited their willingness to meet increased need, state and local governments have begun in the 1980s to seek new ways to finance and deliver medical care to the uninsured, especially those who are poor. Policy makers have recognized the need to segregate the uninsured population into manageable segments, such as workers, the unemployed, mothers and children, the elderly, the homeless, and the "uninsurable" chronically ill.[87,88] The public sector has also proposed that the government and the private sector cooperate in financing care. Some policy makers are also examining the potential of more cost-effective delivery approaches, such as competitively bid contracts or risk-sharing arrangements. Experiments of this type show promise, but before creative, cost-effective systems can deliver services to the uninsured poor, stable and adequate means of financing care for those who are indigent must be available. Providers may accept public grants to defray some of the costs of unsponsored care, but it is unlikely that they will bid to provide such care unless the payment they receive covers at least their marginal costs.

Policy makers are attracted to risk-sharing arrangements, such as HMOs, because HMOs have been demonstrated to save between 10 and 40% of the cost of care per subscriber, primarily through reduced hospitalization and increased ambulatory care.[89] To be cost-effective, these organizations must control hospital care, and the government must be willing to fund a benefit package that includes at least basic preventive and primary services if it wishes to use HMOs for the uninsured. Adequate funding is necessary to ensure that providers are willing to share in the financial risk of managing care for poor enrollees. Because many state and local indigent care programs are not now funded to cover basic benefits, they may have difficulty implementing meaningful and innovative delivery approaches. An adequately financed program is important to meet the current need and to provide sufficient resources to develop new delivery systems for the uninsured poor.

This chapter examines state initiatives for the uninsured from the perspective of available sources of financing rather than subcategories of the population to be served. The first question policy makers, especially legislators, generally ask is "Where can we find dollars to pay for health care for indigents?" Although targeting groups of people who need assistance is an equally important next step in exploring the issue of indigent care, it is generally subordinate to locating sources of funding. Often, in fact, the most politically accessible funding mechanisms effectively determine the populations that will be covered. Whether or not this is the most logical approach to policy making, it is so pervasive that it guides the following discussion.

Improving access to medical care for the poor and uninsured requires a commitment to increased funding. As hospital cost shifting illustrates, for indigent health care there is no "free lunch."* Virtually all care provided to the uninsured poor is paid for directly

---

*Because it is unclear whether and to what extent physicians raise charges to cover costs of their charity care, it may be that there is at least a "free hors d'oeuvre" for some of this care. There may be, of course, an economic opportunity cost to society for even this care.

through taxes imposed on various populations or indirectly through higher hospital charges to self-pay patients or higher insurance premiums to purchasers of health insurance. State and local governments seeking new means of financing indigent care have recognized this limit to the number of revenue sources and have attempted to share the financing burden among various levels of government and specific portions of the private sector, particularly hospitals. It is useful to categorize financing sources as government tax revenues or private sector contributions, recognizing, of course, that all taxes derive from private sector sources but that the distribution of the tax burden varies. For instance, state governments can impose income or excise (sales) taxes, which fall on different tax payers. Local governments are generally supported by property taxes. When the public imposes medical care financing or delivery obligations on the private sector, these costs are borne by insurance subscribers and consumers of other goods and services.

Public Sector Financing Sources

Federal Government Sources

Federal government financing of indigent care is attractive because of the federal government's broad general revenue tax base, which is generally recognized as progressive and which may distribute the tax burden more equitably than before under the 1986 tax reform law. Because of its budget deficits, however, the federal government seems an unlikely source to tap for medical care financing. Indeed, no sweeping proposals for a publicly funded national health program are being debated in Congress in 1988, although Representative Dellums (D-CA) reintroduced his "Health Service" bill and Senator Kennedy (D-MA) is holding hearings in the 100th Congress on a series of proposals described in Chapter 4. Discussions have turned instead to Medicare coverage of "catastrophic" health care costs for the elderly and to some additional Medicaid expansions. The Reagan administration has regularly proposed Medicaid caps and other health care cutbacks that worry state legislators.[90] Nevertheless, the federal health budget, including funding for Medicaid, Medicare, community health centers, veterans' programs, block grants, and a variety of categorical health programs, totals more than $100 billion, having grown steadily in recent years, but now subject to deficit reduction pressures. Furthermore, under Medicare's prospective payment system (diagnosis related groups, DRGs), hospitals with a disproportionate share of charity care are entitled to receive an additional Medicare subsidy. Unfortunately, administration of this provision has been a source of contention among hospitals, the Health Care Financing Administration, and Congress, but if the statute were properly implemented, it would assist individual hospitals with large Medicaid and unsponsored care burdens.

Because of Medicaid's generous federal matching formula, several states have recognized the potential for sharing their indigent care financing burdens with the federal government by expanding state Medicaid programs' eligibility and services to cover more of the otherwise uninsured poor. In a remarkable about-face from Medicaid reductions in the late 1970s, from 1981 through 1987 three dozen states added optional eligibility groups, and many others added covered benefits. Medicaid expansions first became popular when in 1980 Congress allowed states to cover children and pregnant women under "limited medically needy" programs, without also requiring them to cover the medically needy elderly, blind, and disabled. Georgia, Iowa, Mississippi, Oregon, South Carolina, and Texas adopted such programs. Florida and New Jersey adopted full medically needy programs in 1985. Despite the addition of new Medicaid groups, from 1979 to 1983, total enrollment of noninstitutional Medicaid beneficiaries increased only about 1%.[91] Program expansions through 1983 apparently just compensated for the reductions of the late 1970s and early 1980s. Many states have added maternal and child coverage since 1985, which should augment enrollment. Medicaid expansion does offer potential for significant future increases in coverage of target groups.

It is noteworthy that most of the states that expanded Medicaid are Southern. Compared with programs of Northern states, their programs have been traditionally more limited, covering fewer options and allowing more opportunity for growth. Furthermore, Southern states receive above-average federal matching rates (the highest currently is 78%), which makes Medicaid expansion especially attractive in the South. These states have been able to share with the federal government costs that the public or private sectors were already bearing to a large extent.

The flexibility to cover pregnant women and children has also encouraged Medicaid expansion, because medical care for these populations is demonstrably cost-effective[14] and because low birth weight and its attendant economic and human costs have been recognized as a particularly pressing policy issue in the South.[92]

Because more than half the states did not cover all potentially eligible Medicaid groups in 1986,[56] expanding Medicaid is a viable strategy that is being seriously considered. The new opportunity to increase eligibility ceilings is also an attractive option. In 1987, 20 states extended Medicaid eligibility to young children and pregnant women with incomes between previous state levels and the federal poverty level. AFDC income eligibility standards in two-thirds of the states are less than half the poverty line.[56] Raising welfare eligibility levels would immediately increase Medicaid enrollment as well as improve living standards for the working poor. Texas and South Carolina are among the few states to raise these levels as an explicit strategy to improve indigent medical care.

Expanding Medicaid is only a partial solution to the problem of medical care for the poor in view of Medicaid's categorical limitations.[59] Furthermore, several states that have added medically needy and other care groups have had difficulty enrolling the target populations. In Florida and South Carolina, only 10 to 15% of the estimated eligible people have enrolled under the enlarged programs. Special outreach efforts are needed to enlist these groups of working poor.

State Government Sources

In seeking new financing for indigent medical care programs, some states have been willing to expand general revenue budgets, but most have looked for new tax bases or taxes that can be designated for indigent care. The most popular approach has been the hospital tax, pioneered by Florida in 1984. The revenue from this 1.5% tax on hospitals' net revenues forms a pool of about $100 million annually, which is designed to fund the state's expanded Medicaid program and some ambulatory care at selected local health clinics. (Because of lower-than-expected Medicaid enrollment, this pool developed a large surplus, which brought calls to modify the tax or redirect its distribution.) West Virginia and South Carolina adopted hospital taxes in 1985, the former to assist in funding Medicaid and the latter to fund (in combination with a county appropriation) charity care provided by hospitals. Several state legislatures considered similar hospital taxes in 1986 and 1987.* In some of these proposals, for-profit hospitals, which pay income and property taxes, would be credited for the value of such taxes.

Hospital taxes are seen as a politically expedient source of new government revenue and also as a relatively simple means of leveling the playing field for competition by equalizing the charity care burden among hospitals so that none bears a disproportionate share. These taxes are not perfect answers to policy problems, however. As a tax base, hospital revenues are far less equitable than general public income taxes. They are often criticized as a tax on the sick, and they may be borne disproportionately by the relatively small number of uninsured patients who pay full charges. However, they are passed on to all insured people in the form of higher premiums and therefore merely transform the hidden tax of cost shifting into a somewhat more explicit, but still indirect, tax.

Hospital taxes are also a crude means of distributing the costs of indigent care among hospitals. Programs that fund only Medicaid from these taxes do nothing to meet the costs of the poor who are ineligible for Medicaid. Furthermore, the relationship between Medicaid and charity care is not direct and changes over time. Many hospitals with substantial indigent care loads also have large Medicaid populations, but the reverse is not always true. Private hospitals, for instance, may increase Medicaid caseloads while decreasing free care, leaving public hospitals a greater share of charity care but decreased numbers of Medicaid patients.[69] Paying hospitals through the Medicaid program may therefore have little impact on their unsponsored care burdens. Systems that pool these tax revenues and redistribute them according to actual charity care load are more likely to reduce the competitive disadvantage of providing unsponsored care, but if the total amount of such care in a state costs more than the revenues generated, some hospitals will continue to bear an uneven share of charity service.

---

*Current information on proposed state bills and recently enacted legislation on indigent care can be obtained from Debra Lipson and Dick Merrit, Intergovernmental Health Policy Project, 2100 Pennsylvania Avenue, NW, Washington, DC 20037, (202) 872–1445, or from David Landes and Martha King, National Conference of State Legislatures, 1050 17th Street, Denver, CO 80265, (303) 623–7800.

In the late 1980s, states also adopted or considered other taxing authorities. Iowa uses insurance premium taxes and Ohio uses motor vehicle license taxes to fund health care for the poor. Lottery funds in Pennsylvania support pharmaceutical services for the elderly. Alaska and Minnesota increased their cigarette taxes to fund health programs, and other states have considered such legislation. A South Carolina bill proposed but not enacted would have created a state lottery with funds earmarked for indigent care. A 1987 Missouri proposal would have earmarked income tax for a statewide health insurance program. Oklahoma authorizes an income tax refund "check off" into a state indigent care pool. Bills introduced in Oklahoma, Pennsylvania, and Tennessee would have dedicated insurance premium taxes for indigent medical care. Legislators generally dislike earmarked taxes because they set a precedent targeted by other interest groups seeking to fund pet projects, such as environmental protection or child abuse prevention programs. Nevertheless, the future is likely to bring variations on this theme of devising new sources of public revenue through excise and provider taxes.

Local Government Sources

The precise extent of local financing of indigent medical care is unknown, but given the large number of states in which counties or cities are solely responsible for such care, local funding is undoubtedly substantial. The burden on local governments is especially heavy because their primary revenue source is property tax, which may be regressive and is politically difficult to increase.

Legislation in many states permits one or more counties to form hospital or health care districts governed by elected officials with authority to levy property taxes. Many rural hospitals in Colorado and Texas, for instance, are financed and operated by such districts. In some states, local governments can impose sales or income taxes. One Colorado county applies its sales tax to support a county-operated hospital and nursing home. Such earmarked local funds appear to be rare and are an unlikely source of future revenues. Most local governments must have voter approval before imposing or earmarking such taxes. Considering the steady growth of medical care expenditures, voters might hesitate to approve new taxes for indigent care. Local funding sources should therefore be considered limited and unlikely to increase significantly. In recognition of the indigent care financing burden on local government, South Dakota and Texas enacted legislation to protect counties from large costs for individual patients: The states will pay any costs of care above $20,000 or $30,000 per patient, respectively.[67]

Private Sector Financing Sources

Many states have chosen to share indigent care financing with the private sector by imposing indigent care obligations directly on hospitals and insurers, although acknowledging that this imposition indirectly taxes people buying health care services. Current proposals have focused on hospitals, which provide the largest share of indigent care and are easier to regulate than individual providers, such as physicians. Theoretically, states could mandate physicians and other professionals to provide charity care. Massachusetts, which requires physicians to accept Medicare assignment as a condition of the state medical license, has taken such a step. Since that effort was upheld in court in 1987, Vermont and Connecticut have enacted similar mandates, and other states may follow.

Health Care Providers

The first explicit government requirement that hospitals provide charity care was the provision in the federal Hill-Burton Hospital Construction Act of 1946[93] that as a quid pro quo for hospital and nursing home construction loans and grants, recipients would have to provide "a reasonable volume of service to persons unable to pay therefor." Hill-Burton funds flowed for 25 years, however, before this statutory mandate was enforced through litigation. In 1970, the federal government defined the free-service obligation to be 3% of each grantee institution's annual operating costs for 20 years and also mandated that the facility participate in Medicare and Medicaid in perpetuity.

Although Hill-Burton free care has been an important source of access for the poor in the past decade, it has not provided new funds for several years, and current hospital obligations are scheduled to terminate in the 1990s. It does provide, however, an important precedent for similar government requirements by states and municipalities. States that authorize tax-exempt hospital capital financing, for instance, could impose charity care obligations as a prerequisite for financing approval. And states could make affirmative use of tax law by conditioning hospital tax exemptions on provision of specific amounts of charity care.

A number of states have long obligated hospitals with emergency rooms to provide emergency care to patients, regardless of ability to pay,[72] and such requirements have often been reinforced by malpractice liability awards. Despite such mandates, however, hospital "dumping" of emergency charity patients onto the doorsteps of other, usually public, institutions without stabilizing the patients or making referral arrangements has been widespread.[8] Effective in 1986, Congress prohibited this practice for all hospitals participating in Medicare (virtually all U.S. hospitals) for all—not just Medicare—patients. This far-reaching federal law prohibits transferring an emergency patient (defined to include a woman in labor) unless his or her condition has been stabilized or a physician certifies that the move would better serve the patient. In either event, the receiving hospital must agree to the transfer. Both the government and private parties may enforce this law through injunctions and civil penalties. This Medicare amendment was adopted shortly after Texas enacted the first explicit antidumping law in 1985. Seven other states have enacted similar laws, and four more have considered such legislation. The Texas statute was upheld in 1987 in federal court against a challenge by physicians required by a hospital to provide free care as a condition of their staff privileges.[94]

No states have mandated hospital charity care as a condition of licensure, although Maine adopted regulations under its rate-setting program in 1987. Other states are considering wide-ranging proposals. In 1985 the Texas legislature rejected a bill that would have required as a condition of obtaining a state license to operate that a hospital provide at least 3% of its costs (the Hill-Burton formula) as direct charity care or as cash into a pool for distribution to other hospitals. Several other states have developed similar proposals, called hospital "fair share" or "care or share" models. Although these proposals vary, they all would involve designating local hospital service areas, determining the overall level of hospital charity care provided in each area, and apportioning the fair share of such charity service for each hospital, based on gross revenues, patient load, or other measures. The actual amount of charity service, valued by a common scale, such as cost, and adjusted for case severity, would be periodically tallied. Hospitals providing less than their fair share "would pay cash into a pool that would be redistributed to the hospitals who had provided more than their share.[95] In 1987 Nevada enacted a variant of this model, requiring all hospitals either to provide free care to the poor equal to 0.6% of net revenues or to pay this amount to counties to fund indigent care. The New Jersey legislature amended its rate-setting system in 1987 to create a similar pool, funded by a uniform 10% assessment on all hospital rates. Hospitals that do not spend all of their assessment on charity care remit the excess to the pool, which is distributed to hospitals whose charity service exceeds this amount.

These models can be more sensitive than fixed taxes, such as Florida's, to actual levels of charity care in a community and are a more direct redistributive mechanism. They should therefore better promote equality among indigent care providers. But the more these programs vary by geography, case mix, and the value of each provider's charity care, the more complex they are to administer, which may explain why several programs have been proposed from 1985 to 1987 without legislative success.

All programs requiring hospitals or other medical care providers to deliver uncompensated care institutionalize cost shifting, because they provide no additional source of revenue for that care.* For community hospitals providing small levels (3 to 8%) of charity care, the marginal cost of additional charity is actually much less than its valuation based on full charges, and it could easily be sustained, especially if distributed equally among all such institutions.[79] In general, however, this approach is an indirect tax that would be more equitably borne if it were directly imposed by government. Nevertheless, in the short run hospital obligations are seen as a realistic source of financing that is more politically popular than new taxes—especially in states with hospital lobbies that are not very powerful. The use of hospital obligations may also have the long-term advantage of developing a broader constituency

---

*Although Hill-Burton did provide construction dollars, part of which were to be repaid in the form of charity care, the obligation was enforced long after most grants had been awarded and spent. Therefore, Hill-Burton charity care was also financed by raising prices for paying patients.

for a more comprehensive, publicly funded solution to the problem of financing medical care for the uninsured.

Employers

In the private sector, the most pervasive source of funds for medical care is private insurance. Expanding insurance options is therefore another means of increasing private sector funding of care for the currently uninsured. In the United States, employers are the source of most private health, which they offer and, to a great extent, finance. The major incentive for providing this benefit, besides employee goodwill and productivity, is the tax deductibility of health insurance premiums. The federal government supports this employer subsidy with more than $30 billion in foregone general revenues. Because almost 90% of the uninsured are attached to the work force as employees or their dependents, states have recognized that increasing private workplace insurance could substantially reduce the number of people who are uninsured.

The state of Hawaii mandates that all employers offer insurance to their full-time employees and pay part of the premium. The law exempts from coverage people who are self-employed, employees working fewer than 20 hours per week, students, immigrants, spouses, and dependents. Other states, however, are foreclosed from imposing similar obligations by the U.S. Supreme Court's interpretation of the federal Employee's Retirement Income Security Act (ERISA), which preempts state regulation of employee health and pension plans.[96]

It may be possible to circumvent ERISA by imposing an indigent care tax on employers who do not offer employee health insurance. In enacting its 1988 "pay or play" program, Massachusetts hopes to avoid the ERISA preemption by imposing a tax that is refundable if employers provide insurance. This far-reaching plan (the first of several "state health insurance" initiatives to be adopted) requires that in 1992 all employers with six or more workers pay a 12% payroll tax on the first $14,000 of wages for employees who work at least 30 hours per week into a state health care financing fund. Employers offering insurance under qualifying private plans may credit premiums against this tax liability. Workers who are not covered through their jobs may participate in a sliding-scale-premium plan financed from this public fund. Health care for the unemployed and other people who are not part of the work force will be provided through the public program, financed by an additional employer tax and the state's hospital rate-setting charity care pool. The public program's size is predicted to diminish as the private sector plans increase coverage.

Thus far, most states exploring this solution to the indigent care dilemma are attempting to develop incentives to assist and encourage employers to offer insurance. The primary reasons cited by employers for not offering health insurance are availability and cost.[30] Until recently, health insurance carriers would rarely write coverage for groups of fewer than eight to ten people, thereby barring very small employers from group coverage. Now, policies are written for groups as small as one, but the premiums are often no lower than they are for individual coverage, so membership in a small group has no particular advantage. Carriers also typically require medical screening for small groups and may disqualify individuals from participation or sometimes refuse to cover the entire group because of the disability or illness of one member. Thus, small groups are treated differently from large ones. (Although most group insurance excludes or limits coverage for preexisting conditions, members of large groups are not disqualified from plan coverage for other health care needs.)

In addition to premium costs, small employers complain of the time costs of selecting a plan: Because policies are changing rapidly, employers often must seek a new plan each year, and cost-containment strategies require employers to become more sophisticated insurance buyers. An employer with a few employees is generally responsible for all the firm's management and operational decisions and is concerned with keeping the business financially sound. Shopping for employee benefits, especially the increasingly complex health benefits, and processing paperwork (including IRS health insurance reporting requirements incorporated into the 1986 Tax Reform Act) demand more time than the employer often feels is cost-effective.

To overcome problems of cost and availability, some small employers have cooperated to form multiple employer trusts, which create larger groups, spreading risk and commanding lower group premiums, and perform tiresome administrative chores, such as selecting and maintaining plans.[97,98] Recognizing that reducing premiums and minimizing paperwork will induce employers to offer insurance, a few states are beginning to devise programs for affordable insurance for small employers.

Several such initiatives are developing under 1986–1989 grants from the Robert Wood Johnson Foundation's Health Care for the Uninsured program. For instance, the state of Arizona is offering small employers the opportunity to buy coverage from the variety of prepaid health plans participating in the Arizona Health Care Cost Containment System (AHCCCS). These plans are selected by the state on the basis of competitive bid, and premiums are expected to be lower than those in the current private insurance market.[98,99] The state of Wisconsin intends to evaluate multiple employer trusts to determine whether to promote them actively among small businesses.[98,99] Two public hospitals in Denver are collaborating with an insurance carrier to offer high-deductible, low-premium coverage for employees of small firms.[98,100] The state of Michigan is developing a public insurance program with low premiums for recently employed former welfare recipients.[98,100] Because loss of Medicaid and the difficulty of obtaining private insurance are major disincentives to leave welfare, the state hopes to ease the transition to permanent employment by offering affordable health insurance.

Some small employers assert that the cost of a typical comprehensive group policy, $60 to $125 per person per month, is prohibitive but that a premium of $25 to $45 is affordable. Once a group is large enough to spread risk broadly, the only other means of reducing premiums are to increase up-front costs to subscribers through high deductibles and coinsurance (ie, offer a catastrophic policy); impose utilization controls; require risk sharing or case management; negotiate fee discounts with providers; or eliminate expensive benefits, such as mental health or hospital care.

Once-prevalent hospitalization (essentially catastrophic) policies have become unfashionable but may regain popularity among relatively healthy young people who want protection against unexpected, but increasingly expensive, hospitalization.[101] HMOs and other cost-controlling plans have not generally served small employers, but Arizona's experiment is designed to offer such risk-sharing arrangements to this underserved market. Projects in Utah and Maine will test the cost-saving potential of insurance plans with case management by primary care physicians paid on a fee-for-service basis.[98,100] Policies covering only ambulatory care and including preventive services to reduce the need for later institutionalization have not generally been marketed in the past* but might be attractive to families with small children. Subscribers would not anticipate needing hospitalization and would have to rely on hospital charity if they did require such care. Such plans would be difficult to design in states with many mandated insurance benefits (such as mental health and substance abuse treatment). Whether small employers and their employees will be able to afford these insurance products and whether they will find the policy limits unattractive are the unresolved questions these experiments may answer.

Increases in the number of small employers who offer their employees insurance can be expected to raise consumer prices for the products and services sold by these businesses. What is particularly confounding is why one-half to two-thirds of small employers offer insurance whereas similarly matched employers are unable or unwilling to do so.[30] Small employers that do provide this benefit have higher costs of doing business than their competitors who do not offer insurance, an apparent disadvantage. It is therefore unclear how a significant increase in workplace insurance coverage among small firms would affect society overall, particularly because employees would probably be expected to contribute part of the premiums. Furthermore, reducing hospitals' unsponsored care would lower costs to payers and should partially offset consumer price increases or redistribute the costs among products.

In the past few years, the business community in several states and localities has generated legislative action on health care for the uninsured. Business interest in this issue derives primarily from concern over rising medical care expenditures (including cost shifting) and a determination to contain them through a competitive marketplace. Businesses have also recognized the need to share the indigent care burden more equitably among providers so that the marketplace can function both efficiently and fairly.[102,103]

---

*Blue Cross of Western Pennsylvania has piloted such insurance, at a premium of $20.00 per month, for indigent children, whose subscriptions are sponsored by churches and civic groups.

Insurers

A variety of obligations that states impose on health insurers expand opportunities for individuals to obtain or retain insurance. The most traditional of these are conversion and continuation requirements (Table 2.1). In 34 states insurers must allow group subscribers to convert to individual coverage and (usually higher) rates when leaving the group. In 31 states insurers must allow people leaving an employer group to retain their group coverage for some period of time, usually 6 to 18 months. Congress recently mandated (PL 99–272) that employers of 20 or more persons offer continuation for 18 months to terminated employees and 36 months to their widows, divorced or separated spouses, and children. The subscriber, not the employer, pays the premium, which cannot exceed 102% of the per capita premium charged to the group. This requirement applies equally to self-insured and commercially insured firms. Noncompliance disqualifies the employer's entire health insurance plan from tax deductibility.

Insurance continuation and conversion are important protections for insured employees who lose or change employment. The new federal continuation standards should be especially helpful to widows and to divorced people who would be without coverage if their spouses were to die. Nevertheless, to benefit from continuation subscribers must be able to afford the premiums, which may be too expensive for laid-off employees or their spouses.[101] Continuation requirements provide short-term protection—the longer-term unemployed would have to seek more costly individual policy coverage—and they have no effect on the many employees not offered insurance through their workplaces. They are, however, a partial strategy to assist the temporarily unemployed.

An increasingly popular approach to assist the uninsured is the requirement that all insurers participate in risk pools for medically uninsurable people with chronic conditions, such as diabetes, or serious illnesses, such as cancer in remission. A small proportion, between 0.5% and 1%, of the American population is estimated to be medically uninsurable.[104] Many people with AIDS will add to this population. Many uninsurable people have incomes sufficient to pay premiums but find that no one will insure them at any price. Fifteen states have adopted risk pool requirements (Table 2.1) covering subscribers who have been refused coverage by at least one insurer. Insurers must offer coverage with premiums not exceeding 125% to 250% of the rate that would be charged to subscribers of similar age and the same sex but who do not have serious medical problems. Because actual costs of care for risk pool subscribers may be much higher than premiums, most pools operate at a loss and spread additional costs among the participating insurers.[69] Wisconsin and Maine are the only states to subsidize their pools with state funds.

Because few Americans are medically uninsurable and because the poor cannot afford pool premiums, risk pools address a very small part of the problem of the uninsured. They can be useful, however, for people who can afford the coverage. And they can also help small employers offer insurance to employees because risk pools can insure workers whose chronic illness would disqualify not only them but their entire group from commercial coverage. Adopting a risk pool could therefore tie into a state's broader strategy to expand insurance options for small employers.

Risk pools also raise a difficult dilemma because of ERISA. Some courts have held that ERISA prohibits states from requiring that self-insured firms join the pools. Further, risk pool and other requirements, such as mandated benefits and premium taxes, provide a motivation for firms to self-insure and avoid joining the pools. Without full insurer participation, costs are not borne evenly, an increasing concern because nearly half of all group insurance is underwritten by self-insured firms, and the pool for sharing risk continues to diminish.[105]

Despite these disadvantages, the number of states with risk pools doubled from 1985 to 1987. Risk pooling will assume increasing importance as the group insurance market becomes more segmented. HMOs and indemnity carriers are increasingly attempting to enroll healthy people, leaving high-risk subscribers to the older, more comprehensive plans.[105] These strategies, although economically rational, undermine the risk-sharing concept of traditional health insurance and leave high-risk people with higher premiums and diminishing sources of coverage.

Hospital rate setting, though nominally regulation of hospital revenues, is another means of spreading the cost of charity care among all payers: commercial insurers, Blue Cross, self-insured firms, public payers (not Medicare in most states), and self-pay patients. Insurers are required through rate setting to pay a share of the hospitals' bad debt and charity. In some states, rate setting is the financial basis of a revenue pool used to fund indigent care (not necessarily merely uncompensated hospital care).[71] Although it may seem antithetical to discuss rate setting in an era devoted to competition, as of 1987 nine states had mandatory rate-setting systems, including three (Maine, West Virginia, and Wisconsin) that enacted laws since 1985. States with such mandatory programs have experienced hospital expenditures that are two to three percentage points (about 25%) lower than those in other states.[49]

Another insurance regulation approach is to prohibit insurers (other than self-insured firms) from refusing to cover part-time employees (15 to 35 hours per week); New Hampshire recently adopted this approach. (Changes in federal tax law to accomplish the same objective are discussed in Chapter 4.) Although the decision not to cover part-time employees is often made by the employer, the extent to which it is dictated by insurers' policies could be countermanded by state insurance regulation.

Medical Care Consumers

Although uninsured poor consumers cannot be expected to provide a substantial proportion of indigent care financing, many have incomes above the poverty level and could share in the costs of their own care. Indeed, considering the multifaceted approach states are taking to distribute indigent care responsibilities, consumers must contribute directly toward financing this care. Legislators and other groups involved in trying to solve the problem of access also expect consumers to do so. Many small employers require employees to share in the insurance premium. Most public indigent programs require copayment based on ability to pay.

Recent analyses of cost sharing demonstrate its effectiveness in reducing health care utilization and costs, but these and other studies show potentially deleterious effects on the health status of the poor if they delay or forego necessary care because of prohibitive copayment requirements.[106] Requesting that patients with some means share in financing their own care may sensitize them to its costs, but any efforts to collect small copayments beyond the point of service are expensive and may not be worth their cost.

Cost-Effective Delivery Systems

A state or local government that has generated a budget sufficient to fund a reasonable set of basic benefits may look for innovative ways to structure the medical care delivery system to inherently contain expenditures. For instance, if a state indigent care
program includes basic ambulatory and hospital care, it can enroll
eligibles in HMOs or other plans in which providers bear some of
the financial risk for serving a defined population during a specified
period. Half of the states currently enroll Medicaid populations in
HMOs, but these enrollees represent only 5% of those eligible for
Medicaid. Five states (Arizona, California, Illinois, Michigan, and
Wisconsin) account for 80% of Medicaid's HMO enrollment.[107]
Other options used in many state Medicaid programs are partial
capitation (eg, for outpatient care only) or case management by a
primary care physician, which means a physician is paid a fee to
manage the care of a Medicaid patient and to authorize care from
any other provider.

In 1987 the state of Washington enacted a far-reaching law to
pilot test in five communities enrollment of uninsured residents
with incomes under 200% of the poverty level into prepaid health
care delivery plans.[100] Under the Robert Wood Johnson grant program, Michigan, Maine, and Wisconsin will test the feasibility of
enrolling the uninsured poor (general relief recipients and the
working poor) into "managed" health care systems. Wisconsin
plans to pilot a voucher system that would allow employees in firms
without insurance to buy coverage from a group policy meeting
minimum state standards.[99] Michigan is developing a case management system for its general assistance and post-AFDC clients.[100]
Physicians will be paid to oversee and care for a defined population.
Patients, employers, and the state will jointly fund the program.
Bills modeled on Arizona's system to provide prepaid and case-
managed care for the uninsured poor have been introduced in
Alaska and Minnesota.

Some policy makers express concern that the uninsured are an
inherently unstable and transient group that cannot be successfully
enrolled into organized delivery systems. Transience could impose
an especially great burden on the providers that bear risk, because
a minimum enrollment period is usually necessary to stabilize
health status and educate subscribers in how to use these systems.

Although many of the uninsured are employed people who have families and could probably be enrolled in HMOs or other case management arrangements, others are undoubtedly more transient and therefore more difficult to enlist into organized systems. The low-income population includes families whose Medicaid eligibility changes as jobs and income change. For this group, a statewide program that allows retaining eligibility in one plan while the source of payment changes—from Medicaid to employer or state indigent care program and back (such as that contemplated for Wisconsin)—would minimize disruption and encourage enrollees to use the plan appropriately.

Experience in Arizona's Health Care Cost Containment System (AHCCCS) plan underscores the difficulty of enrolling the non-Medicaid poor. AHCCCS was designed to cover all state indigents (formerly served by county programs) through prepaid plans. Care for the categorical groups eligible for Medicaid is financed by the state and federal governments, and counties continue to finance the noncategorical poor. Despite initial difficulties, AHCCCS seems to have overcome problems of contracting with and paying providers. Medicaid AFDC and SSI enrollments are progressing as expected, and analysis suggests that access to care for these groups has improved. But the state has been unable to obtain broad participation by traditional private sector HMOs in its program.[108] Furthermore, one study revealed that more than half of AHCCCS enrollees were refused care by plan providers, possibly because of eligibility confusion or pre-authorization requirements.[109] Given the potential for provider fraud and underservice in prepaid plans,[110] it is especially important to educate consumers to use these plans appropriately and to monitor utilization patterns.

In addition, many of Arizona's non-Medicaid poor, who must enroll themselves without participating directly in the welfare system, appear not to be receiving the benefits available to them. One study showed that the noncategorical (non-Medicaid-eligible) indigent patients who were eligible for AHCCCS were less likely than those who were eligible for AFDC and SSI to be enrolled in AHCCCS and were less likely to report having a usual source of care and to make ambulatory visits. These differences increased as the respondents' reported health status declined.[54] The working poor can be enrolled through the workplace, as intended by Arizona's new initiative, but for the nonworking, nonwelfare poor, an

active recruiting effort is needed to provide the benefit of a prepaid, case-managed system. This objective may be difficult to
achieve.

Cost-Effective Care

Innovative systems for delivering indigent care may be available only in states having comprehensive funding commitments
and many geographically dispersed provider networks. A somewhat more practical, immediately effective approach is financing
cost-effective services for special populations. For example, the interest in improved pregnancy outcomes and early childhood health
has led Congress to expand Medicaid eligibility for pregnant
women and has led several states to adopt specific prenatal care
initiatives. Iowa, whose state-funded indigent program is operated
through the University of Iowa Hospital, is experimenting with a
decentralized system of maternity services provided through local
community hospitals, an approach similar to one adopted in 1979 by
Colorado (the Community Maternity Program).[22] In 1985 Texas enacted legislation to create programs targeting maternal and child
health, including grants for maternal and infant programs in local
communities and for primary care services. Maryland, Massachusetts, Michigan, Minnesota, and New York also adopted statutory
prenatal care programs in 1986 and 1987, and several other states
have introduced similar bills.

Financing cost-effective services should lower medical care
costs in the long term, but it would be inappropriate for government to reduce acute care funding as an immediate cost-saving effort because the financial return from preventive care—the reduced need for acute care—can take many years to materialize.

Conclusion

The many state and local governments now attempting to solve
the problem of access to medical care for the poor and uninsured all
are seeking new financing sources and more cost-effective means to
care for the growing uninsured population. Ultimately, the costs of
care or the consequences of foregone care will be supported by society at large, but the financing burden can be distributed variously—among payers of property, income, or excise taxes; purchasers of medical care and health insurance; purchasers of

employers' goods and services; and the poor themselves. Although a general federal or state income tax financing system would most equitably distribute the cost, political expediency—the need to find the most politically acceptable formula to fund this obligation—often overcomes the search for an equitable taxing mechanism because of the current pressure on the public sector to disperse its indigent care costs. The immediate solution to the problem of the uninsured will be state and municipal attempts to distribute indigent care costs among various public and private sector groups. Although this approach lacks financing equity, it may have the advantage of keeping the issue in public view and generating a large, diverse constituency for broader public financing reform and a national agenda for access to medical care. Options for such a national agenda are the subject of the next chapter.

4

The Unfinished National Agenda for Universal Access to Medical Care

The problem of access to medical care for the poor and uninsured is evidently growing. The number of uninsured Americans may be increasing, a trend that is likely to continue, even in a robust economy, as the country shifts from a manufacturing to a service work force. A greater proportion of the population may also become inadequately insured as employers attempt to control their premium costs by limiting benefits and expanding subscribers' copayments. Even if the percentage of the population that is uninsured or underinsured stabilizes, however, hospitals and other providers will face the need to limit charity care as they attempt to lower costs and prices to compete in the medical care marketplace. The pressure to lower prices is unlikely to diminish, because government and private purchasers will continue to seek ways to lower medical care expenditures. Thus, the question of how to eliminate economic barriers to access to medical care will remain a pressing public policy concern.

More than half of the states and numerous municipalities have studied the problem of indigent care, and many have adopted various approaches to deal with it. In view of these state and local activities, why is a national policy on access to medical care necessary? The simple answer is that the problem is a national one, a fact that Congress acknowledged when it adopted Medicaid and Medicare 20 years ago.

The vast disparities in resources and political commitments among states assure that people with identical economic and health status have entirely different opportunities to obtain needed health care.[59] If medical care is recognized as a human good,[16] not a market commodity, the nation as a whole is obliged to secure for all citizens access to basic medical services. The United States is the only industrialized nation except South Africa with no national health protection program. Furthermore, without an explicit national policy, the nation has, in fact, adopted an implicit one: tax-subsidized private insurance for the middle and upper classes, a reasonably generous public insurance program for many of the poor, but no basic medical care financing protection for about half of the very poor and millions of the near-poor. The policy also makes financially endangered public hospitals the providers of last resort, while permitting most private tax-exempt hospitals to limit their share of charity care to that provided in emergency cases.

Another reason to adopt a national policy on access to medical care is that even if states should assume the primary responsibility to finance and administer programs of care for the poor and uninsured, federal policies, particularly tax and pension laws, now inhibit states' ability to do so effectively. State and local governments have acted because they are, historically and legally, ultimately responsible for the health and welfare of their residents. They cannot wait for federal leadership. But resource limitations impede their ability to solve the indigent care problem, and their legal and practical authority over businesses that employ a large share of the uninsured is limited by federal constraints. Changes in federal law plus additional resources, at the very least, are necessary to permit states to assure access to medical care for their residents.

A national policy does not necessarily require a federally financed and operated national health plan, although that is the most comprehensive and perhaps the most equitable solution to the dilemma. More modest national strategies could invoke tax policy to encourage more employer-sponsored insurance and more hospital charity care. Federal law could also establish a basic minimum program of health care protection that states must guarantee and that could incorporate private and public sector financing and delivery options. Further, federal law could allow states more flexibility to develop indigent care initiatives. This chapter explores the spectrum of approaches for a national policy on access to medical care for the poor and uninsured.

Retain Existing Federal Laws and Programs

To move ahead with new initiatives to expand access to medical care, the nation should strengthen, not undercut, the effectiveness of existing programs. We must enforce vigorously the recent protection for hospital emergency patients enacted through PL 99–272.[10] In addition to allowing injured patients to sue, the law authorizes the U.S. Justice Department to impose penalties on violators. Public hospitals that receive unauthorized emergency transfers should be encouraged to report such abuses, and violators should be prosecuted. Although this legal mandate is a modest effort to distribute some of the charity care burden among all hospitals, it is an important measure to ensure that the private sector participates more equitably than before in financing indigent medical care.

Also enforceable is the 1983 requirement of PL 97–35 that Medicare make additional payments to hospitals serving a disproportionate number of the poor. The federal Health Care Financing Administration has been loathe to apply this mandate, despite several explicit congressional directives and a federal court order. Payments to these providers could be an important source of extra funding that can help stabilize them in the face of declining private revenues.

Perhaps most important is continued adequate funding of Medicaid. The Reagan administration's annual budget proposals through fiscal year 1988 routinely requested a cap on the federal government's share of Medicaid financing, based on the contribution of an earlier year with an allowance for inflation in medical expenditures. Thus, Medicaid would have become a block grant, rather than an open-ended federal entitlement program. States would therefore have had either to cut eligibility or to finance a larger share of Medicaid if the federal inflation factor were underestimated or if eligibility expanded, as it might during an economic recession. States would also have had no incentive to add new services or eligibility groups. And although the cap was purportedly designed to encourage state efficiencies, it would have penalized states that had recently actively sought to contain Medicaid expenditures: These states would have had less opportunity to save through future efficiencies, compared with the less provident states that had not yet exploited cost-control strategies.

This is a particularly inappropriate time to discourage adding new eligibility groups, given the significantly expanded Medicaid eligibility option that Congress enacted through PL 99–509 (1986), PL 100–203 (1987), and PL 100–360 (1988). The very threat of a limit on federal participation is effective despite being annually rejected by Congress. Many state legislatures fear the risk of reduced federal funding that states would face with such a cap; several have recently refused to expand their Medicaid programs by adding optional eligibility groups and benefits. Although this rationale may seem a convenient excuse for inaction, particularly in light of the many Medicaid expansions that Congress has enacted since 1981, the risk is a very real concern. Congress can reassure reluctant state legislatures only by consistently affirming Medicaid's value and longevity as well as the federal commitment to shared financing.

Augment Revenue Sources

It may be unrealistic to request that Congress provide additional dollars from the tight federal budget to the states for indigent care, especially as other revenue-sharing funds are threatened. Nevertheless, there is potential for states to benefit from changes in federal tax policy. For instance, when the federal cigarette tax was scheduled to expire in 1984, several states planned to augment their own tobacco taxes to capitalize on consumers' expectation of a certain tax level. Some states planned to use this additional excise tax for indigent health care programs. Unfortunately for these states, the federal government decided to retain its federal tax.

Given the federal deficit, the opportunities to pick up an expiring federal tax may be few, but they should be considered when the federal tax policy is discussed. Increasing provincial taxing authority was the primary means by which Canada encouraged all provinces to adopt public hospital insurance in 1966. A potential windfall has existed since 1986 in states with income tax laws that mirror the federal system. Because several personal tax deductions were eliminated in the 1986 federal tax law, income taxes in these states will increase automatically unless tax rates are lowered. States could use this opportunity to increase their tax revenues without explicitly raising taxes. The demand to return these "extra" dollars to the taxpayers may make it difficult to retain the revenue increase, but if states can keep even part of this windfall, they may be able to increase revenues enough to finance needed improvements in their indigent care programs. Of course, medical care for the poor must compete for these limited dollars with other state-funded programs, such as education and highway construction.

Change Federal Laws

Change Income Tax Laws

The federal government has advanced many of its social policies through the income tax laws. Prime examples of fostering a socially desired objective are the exclusions from employee income of both employer-paid health insurance premiums[111] and benefits paid under health plans,[112] both part of the Internal Revenue Code since 1954. Health plan benefits paid in pre-tax dollars have added economic value to an employee, and this value increases with the employee's marginal tax rate.[113]

Change Requirements for Tax Deductibility of Premiums. Employers deduct their share of the employee health plan premiums they pay.[114] But tax deductibility is limited to qualified plans, which means, for instance, that plans offered by firms with more than 20 employees must give terminated employees and their dependents, widows, and divorced spouses the opportunity to continue their group insurance for up to 18 and 36 months, respectively. By changing the definition of a qualified plan, as it did in PL 99–272, Congress has immense influence on the design of employee health insurance, but it has not frequently exercised this influence. A particular advantage to using the tax code is that it applies to self-insured employers as well as employers using traditional carriers to underwrite insurance risk.

A number of other tax law changes could be included in a federal policy to increase access to health care. Requiring that a plan cover part-time workers and dependents or that an employer pay at least part of an employee's or dependent's premium could help but might also have untoward effects. Changes to Section 89 of the Internal Revenue Code require employers with insurance to offer benefits to people working at least 17.5 hours per week, although the extent of benefits may differ. These requirements will be interpreted in forthcoming IRS rules.[115] Because employees working fewer than 35 hours per week constitute a sixth of the uninsured population,[25] this change may cover many of the uninsured. The tax revisions could, however, be counterproductive if they discourage part-time employment opportunities or induce small employers to drop health insurance entirely because of cumbersome federal reporting requirements under the new law.[115] The effects of potential income tax policy changes should be studied so this powerful incentive is used to provide the greatest social good: health protection for the largest number of American workers through group plans, without loss of employment opportunities for low-wage or part-time workers.

Uninsured dependents of uninsured workers constitute almost 25% of the uninsured population. Another 10 to 12% of the uninsured are dependents of workers with insurance,* most of whom could insure their families if they could afford their share of the premiums. To help these uninsured groups, Congress could mandate that a qualified plan must have dependent coverage available and that employers pay at least part of the premiums for such coverage. The requirement for dependent coverage would not disrupt current benefit arrangements because most plans now cover dependents.**

Requiring employers to contribute to premiums, however, could have an adverse impact on small firms, which are most likely

---

*Personal communication, Alan Monheit, National Center for Health Services Research.

**It has been suggested that "dependent" could be defined to include separated spouses, foster children, and elderly relatives, although such extensions strain the concept of workplace insurance. These extensions would be administratively complex and might lead to adverse selection.[101]

to employ the uninsured. Also, more than half of the employed uninsured have incomes in excess of twice the poverty level, and policies to assist the poor who are uninsured should not provide a windfall to people who are able to afford insurance were it offered. The impact of a mandated employer contribution should therefore be studied to determine whether such a requirement would be counterproductive. Furthermore, any tax law changes that induce greater employee coverage will necessarily reduce tax collections, which will be difficult to justify given the current emphasis on deficit reduction. However, having employers (and their customers), employees, and the federal budget share the costs of insuring some of the currently uninsured may provide the best immediate solution to the problem of financing care for the uninsured.

Retain Tax Deductions but Consider Tax Caps. Because health insurance has become an expected employee benefit, it is difficult to know the extent to which its tax deductibility influences employers' decisions to provide it. Some firms would undoubtedly continue to offer insurance regardless of the tax incentive. Furthermore, this incentive has not been great enough to induce a large proportion of small employers to offer health insurance. Nevertheless, as a matter of medical care access policy, it would be counterproductive to abandon the tax deductibility of health insurance premiums at a time when we want to provide more coverage for the working poor.

Most proposals to change the business tax deduction and employee tax exclusion for health insurance have not suggested eliminating this tax treatment entirely,* but have recommended either taxing as income part of the benefit paid to employees or allowing the deduction for only a certain amount of the employer's monthly premium cost. For instance, the Reagan administration proposed taxing the first $10 per month of employee health benefits to raise medical care cost-consciousness in employees. This proposal was never seriously considered; it not only ill serves its stated purpose but might have the unintended consequence of inducing greater

---

*Enthoven has proposed eliminating tax deductibility and exclusion of health benefits in favor of a national program of tax credits for part of the cost of the least expensive comprehensive plan. This approach would encourage price competition among plans and equalize the tax subsidy among income groups.[113]

use of medical care services by people who feel they have paid for them.

The tax cap proposal is more rational and merits more serious attention. The administration suggested that employers be allowed to deduct no more than $840 per year for individual coverage and $2,100 for family coverage rather than the unlimited premium allowed under current law. Advocates of medical care competition support this change, arguing that limitless deductibility of premiums encourages coverage for services that are not always needed and provides first-dollar coverage (no enrollee cost sharing), which reduces cost-consciousness among enrollees. These observers assert that employees wanting extra benefits should have to buy them with after-tax dollars. Proponents of the plan also hope that limiting premium deductions would lead to more cost-effective plan options becoming available.[37] The tax cap amounts were designed to cover the cost of moderately comprehensive plans with some co-payment by enrollees. The cap was estimated to reduce premiums between $3 and $6 million per year and add more than $3 billion per year to federal revenues. Opponents, including organized labor, health care providers, and the insurance industry, have so far successfully challenged the tax cap proposal as an erosion of hard-won employee benefits and a diminution of important protection against the financial risk of uncovered medical expenses.

Objectively, however, the plan is unlikely to reduce major medical coverage that insures against high-cost but low-probability illness. Analysts of current health plan costs believe the cap would eliminate the deductibility of discretionary benefits, such as vision and dental care, rather than that of hospital and physician care.[37] Insuring for low-cost, predictable, and relatively discretionary services has become the routine method of payment for these services, and such insurance has increased access to and use of such care. But it is not consistent with the traditional premise of insurance: protection against unexpected, costly, and unlikely events.

Eliminating first-dollar coverage can encourage cost-consciousness,[116] but the effects of cost sharing on low-income workers may be adverse[106] and should therefore be addressed by tax rebates or other public assistance for the poor and near-poor. Another concern raised by tax cap opponents is that the proposal does not consider geographic differences in medical care costs or risk factors, such as age and health status.

A tax cap should not be dismissed categorically, however, if it generates additional tax revenues that could be applied to assist the poor and near-poor to purchase insurance or to pay cost sharing to improve their access to needed care. The capped amounts should be carefully set to include the cost of an adequate plan, such as an HMO, and indexed to medical care prices. Furthermore, any tax cap proposal should be promoted as a revenue-raising measure, not as an inducement for behavioral changes.

Reform the Tax Exemption for Donations to Hospitals.   A major incentive for individual and business contributions to charitable causes is the tax deductibility of these donations. To qualify for such favored tax status, organizations must be both nonprofit (under state corporations law) and tax exempt (under the Internal Revenue Code). The major tax exemption for such groups is defined in Internal Revenue Code section 501(c)(3), which specifies requirements for a charitable purpose and activity. The IRS has long held that hospitals and other nonprofit health providers meet the test of being charitable without regard to the amount of free care that they provide. The U.S. Supreme Court upheld this loose interpretation of existing tax law in 1976.[117,118] Congress could, however, mandate explicit amounts of charity care that hospitals must provide to qualify for this tax status. (State courts have varied in interpreting state tax exemption laws to require that hospitals demonstrate certain amounts of charitable service to claim the tax exemption.[74,75]) Such a federal tax law change could induce more hospitals to provide a specific amount of charity care and partially redistribute the charity burden. Even were this incentive unsuccessful, the government would at least regain tax revenue that had been previously lost to the thwarted public purpose of hospitals' charity care.

Change ERISA

The Employee's Retirement and Income Security Act (ERISA) seriously limits the ability of states to regulate health insurance. Because the courts have interpreted ERISA to preempt state regulation of employer health plans,[96] states cannot require that self-insured employers offer insurance to employees, provide any particular set of benefits, or participate in risk-sharing arrangements, such as risk pools for the uninsurable. Nor can states tax the "premiums" paid by self-insured firms. Because states may impose requirements on traditional insurance carriers, employers are not only unregulated but encouraged to self-insure to avoid the cost of providing mandatory benefits and paying premium taxes.

Amending ERISA to allow states to impose requirements on self-insured employers could provide the flexibility states need to address appropriately the problem of the working uninsured. For example, 15 states have enacted risk pool legislation without including self-insured firms, and it is likely that many other states would set up risk pools if they could broaden participation.

States with a large number of uninsured workers and small employers are not especially likely to require business to provide insurance. As experience in Hawaii demonstrates, state regulation might be most feasible where it is least needed. Most workers in Hawaii were insured before the state law (which Congress exempted from the ERISA preemption) took effect.[119] However, authorizing states to mandate coverage and to set minimum acceptable benefits would allow them to meet their unique local needs and political realities. States wishing to adopt such mandates would have to confront several difficult policy issues, such as the treatment of part-time, temporary, and transient employees and the potential adverse and differential effects on some small businesses. These problems are not insurmountable, however, and Hawaii's experience can guide other states. For instance, Hawaii established a fund to assist small businesses to finance insurance, but the fund has rarely been used.[119]

The states of Massachusetts and Minnesota have promoted amending ERISA, and the subject has been widely discussed, because the ERISA preemption has been recognized as a barrier to effective state control over the issue of the working uninsured.[25,84,103,120] Opposition to changing ERISA comes from such predictable sources as private business. Surprisingly, some members of organized labor are also concerned that this approach intrudes on its power to negotiate employee health benefits and provides a precedent for other more serious limitations that might compromise ERISA's broad protection of employee benefits.

Reform Medicaid

One obvious approach to improving financial access to medical care is to expand Medicaid, the nation's major means of financing care for the poor, to overcome its many categorical and income limitations. As discussed in Chapter 2, the 1986 and 1987 Budget Reconciliation Acts (PL 99-509 and PL 100-203) and the 1988 Medicare catastrophic law (PL 100-360) represent an important effort to improve access by breaking the historic link between Medicaid and welfare programs. Nevertheless, Medicaid still entirely omits coverage of most parents in two-parent families, single people, and childless couples. Furthermore, the only groups that may be covered up to the federal poverty level are young children, pregnant women, the elderly, and the disabled, and coverage for people up to 185% of the poverty level is available only for pregnant women and children up to age 1.

Statutory changes since 1981 have added several new mandatory eligibility groups as well as optional groups, but a large number of states have not taken advantage of the law's options. For instance, 18 states do not cover children under age 18 in poor (AFDC income level) two-parent families, 16 do not have a general medically needy program at all, and 13 do not cover women and children as medically needy.[56] Although federal eligibility improvements are encouraging, especially in the face of budget reduction efforts, Medicaid is far from providing health protection for all the poor.

In the past 10 years, there have been a number of proposals to expand and reform Medicaid, proposals ranging from mandating state coverage of currently optional groups, to dividing the program into different eligibility and service components, to total federalization.[59,121] In 1983 a study group composed of nine state Medicaid agency directors proposed a Medicaid reform plan that would have split the current program into two parts: one to cover primary care for all the poor and the other to cover long-term health and social services for the elderly and disabled.[58,63] This task force reasoned that the current Medicaid program cannot achieve the inconsistent objectives of financing and delivering care to two very disparate groups—families with children and people who are functionally, physically, or mentally impaired. Because types of care and delivery approaches differ dramatically for these groups, the task force proposed treating them separately.

The proposed primary care program would be administered by the federal government and financed with state and federal funds and would provide standard inpatient and outpatient benefits and a uniform national eligibility level for all the poor, regardless of family or health status. (This concept is similar to the Family Health Insurance Plan proposed in 1974 by the Nixon administration as an adjunct to a broader welfare reform initiative.) Although budget limits would prohibit setting initial eligibility at the poverty level, proponents hoped that eligibility would eventually reach such a standard. The purpose of the primary care program would be to break the health-welfare connection, establish a uniform national program to eliminate interstate disparities in eligibility and benefits, emphasize preventive and primary care, and promote efficient and cost-effective delivery through the use of case managers, prospective payment, and capitation. The study group estimated only modest increases in state and federal funding because cost-containment strategies were projected to save considerable current program dollars.[63]

The continuing care program to provide health and social services to the functionally disabled would be administered by states under general federal guidelines. Each state would set eligibility levels, benefits, and delivery system approaches. Federal funds would be limited to a block grant based on the number of disabled people in the state and the state's poverty level. The state would be expected to integrate social and health services into a spectrum of long-term care, from housing and nutritional assistance, through in-home support and home health care, to nursing home institutionalization. Low-income beneficiaries of this continuing care program would obtain inpatient and ambulatory care through the federal primary care program or Medicare. Thus, these three public financing systems would be complementary and eliminate gaps and duplication among current government programs.[63]

The study group's proposal is commendable as a comprehensive strategy that begins with current programs, addresses some of their greatest weaknesses, and can be improved and refined over time. It also raises many questions: Are the cost savings projections overly optimistic? How quickly could income eligibility levels be raised? Would the poor living in states with especially generous

Medicaid programs be penalized? Or would these states be allowed to supplement the federal medical care program? If these supplemental programs could not receive federal funding, would they maintain their more generous standards? How could the federal program avoid the disincentive for employers to offer and employees to obtain private insurance that might cost them more than participating in the public program? That is, would public financing, even for very low income families, encourage low-wage employers now offering insurance to drop it, increasing the demands on the public program?

Another concern, in view of states' recent experience, is how to increase enrollment by the nonwelfare population. Some proponents of using Medicaid as the foundation of a national medical care financing strategy would allow groups such as the working poor or disabled to "buy-in" to Medicaid, paying income-based premiums. But such a strategy may require overcoming Medicaid's current welfare stigma. Furthermore, any changes in Medicaid must be carefully coordinated with other policies concerning access to medical care, particularly those concerned with private insurance initiatives and hospital charity.

Because nearly half of the Medicaid budget is devoted to long-term care (expenditures that are swiftly rising as the population ages), many proposals to reform the financing and delivery of the nation's long-term care services have been offered. Long-term care insurance, once considered impossible to design and market, is being actively promoted and is developing slowly.[122] Health and Human Services Secretary Otis Bowen's proposal for a national catastrophic health care policy* includes incentives to buy long-term care insurance and to open medical "investment retirement ac-

---

*Although expanding Medicaid is the most direct means of covering additional uninsured poor people, Medicare's coverage limits also call for reform to protect the elderly from unaffordable health care costs. It is in this spirit that in 1988 Congress passed legislation to limit beneficiaries' annual out-of-pocket costs of Medicare-covered hospital services to approximately $2,000 (PL 100–360). This law does not expand Medicare coverage of long-term care, however, and would not assist the large number of elderly people for whom out-of-pocket acute care costs under $2,000 represent more than 15% of their incomes.[123] A discussion of Medicare reform proposals is beyond the scope of this monograph, and this subject has been well treated elsewhere.[38] However, it should be noted that the threat to viability of the Medicare Trust Funds is likely to bring changes in Medicare for reasons other than equity to beneficiaries. What should be avoided in any case is significant compromise to equity, access, and coverage.

counts" for long-term care. Other analysts have proposed a comprehensive long-term care reform strategy, including the foregoing approaches as well as the development of additional social health maintenance organizations and life care communities.[39]

Opponents of proposals to expand Medicaid emphasize the costs of the current program, especially the unanticipated cost increases in the program's early years. But states have learned from their early experience how to control their medical care expenditures through such means as prepayment, capitation, case management, fraud detection, and utilization review. Medicaid budgets have been increasing at about the same rate as other medical care expenditures. States would, of course, like to slow the growth of their Medicaid costs even further. They will undoubtedly seek more cost-containment opportunities. Restricting beneficiaries' freedom of choice to a selected number of cost-effective plans is an increasingly attractive strategy.

Although consumer advocates have previously opposed limiting choice of providers, they may now find this approach more acceptable. In some communities, finding a provider to treat a Medicaid patient is so difficult that no true freedom of choice exists, so requiring a beneficiary to choose a provider may actually increase access. Furthermore, as employers and insurers begin directly or indirectly to limit their enrollees' freedom to choose providers, parallel limits on Medicaid beneficiaries seem to speak less of a two-tiered medical system than economic necessity for all.

The Problem with These Approaches

These three kinds of change in federal law—modification of the tax code and the ERISA law and Medicaid expansion—could, taken together, form the framework of a national policy on medical care access. Such a modest strategy has the advantage of involving the private sector and limiting demands on the federal budget. It is therefore consistent with current congressional debates on access to care.* Any such fragmented approaches have disadvantages, however.

Making Medicaid and Medicare, in expanded form, the cornerstones of a public health insurance system has been argued to be fundamentally inconsistent with a national strategy for access to medical care.[2] Mandating states to cover more eligible groups would at least maintain the congressional momentum of the past 7 years, but this is a slow and piecemeal solution. Federalizing Medicaid would help only a small number of the uninsured and underinsured who face financial access barriers, particularly because a budget-neutral program would cover some new groups but eliminate many now covered. Amending Medicare to limit out-of-pocket costs or to shore up its future revenues is also an incomplete solution to the larger problem of the underinsured elderly. Federal tax law changes would expand some private insurance coverage, but, as noted, might discourage some marginally profitable employers from offering insurance at all. Modifying ERISA to allow states to mandate employment-based insurance or participation in risk pools does not necessarily mean states will adopt such legislation. Political resistance would be strong, especially in states struggling to revitalize their economies and anxious to attract, not repel, new employers. Furthermore, many people left out of the workforce and ineligible for either a nationalized Medicaid program or a state program would remain without medical care financing. The dilemma that such piecemeal solutions always raise is whether it is better to take some small steps to solve part of the problem—provided that they do not create a larger one—or to wait for a longer term and more comprehensive solution to be feasible and acceptable. It would be irresponsible not to assist people in immediate need. Nevertheless, we must eventually develop a longer term strategy to address the problems of access and increasing medical care expenditures.

---

*In 1986 Senator Kennedy introduced legislation (the Improved Access to Health Care Initiative) that would have required states to establish risk pools and subsidize hospital charity care and bad debt, provided federal demonstration projects to develop lower cost insurance approaches for small business, allowed self-employed people to deduct their insurance premiums, and required employers to offer and pay for continuation coverage for laid-off workers and their spouses.[91] Variations of the last two provisions of this bill were enacted in the 1986 Budget Reconciliation Act, PL 99–272.

Essential: A National Health Financing Plan

Congress first entertained a proposal for national health insurance in 1939.[2] The protracted debate over such legislation finally led more than 20 years later to enactment of Medicare and Medicaid. During the 1970s Congress again considered but rejected about two dozen national health plan bills.[2] In 1980 the Carter administration proposed requiring all employers to offer insurance and expanding coverage for the poor. These proposals were seriously considered in Congress but abandoned when the administration changed. After another hiatus, public discussion of a national health care program seems to have reopened. The debates have hardly begun yet, but they will likely focus on two different approaches: a uniform national health insurance system and a federal approach that places responsibility on states to assure medical care financing for their residents.

A Uniform National Health Care Financing Program

Previous bills for national health programs have proposed two divergent models: a social insurance system (like Medicare) that is uniformly financed and administered and nationally mandated, employer-offered, private sector insurance combined with a federal level public program for people not in the workforce. The Dellums bill, proposing a U.S. National Health Service on the British model but regionally administered, has been introduced in every Congress since 1977. This sweeping reform has not generated much support, but it continues to maintain the issue in public view. National proposals that would receive more serious consideration would use the existing private provider network, private insurers as claims payment agents or underwriters, and employers as either purchasers of insurance or financers of a public program through payroll taxes.

Although the public social insurance model is attractive for its universality and comparatively simple administration, it is likely that future national health care financing proposals will include a mandate for employment-based insurance. This is the approach taken by Senators Kennedy and Simon in S. 1265, which passed the Senate Labor and Human Resources Committee in early 1988. A practical rationale for shared public-private sector responsibilities is to limit the portion of the federal budget devoted to medical care.

(In 1977 it would have more than doubled to 22% were a national health insurance program financed through the federal government, even if total expenditures did not increase.[2]) Furthermore, it is hard to ignore workplace-based insurance because it is well established and accepted. If the government assisted marginally profitable employers through risk pools or tax credits, the workplace would provide a stable foundation on which to build a national health care financing program. Tying health benefits to the workplace reinforces the traditional American work ethic. Furthermore, the political power of insurance carriers cannot be overlooked. People who lament abandoning a social insurance approach or retaining the costly private insurance industry may be comforted by Milton Roemer's reminder that most industrialized nations began their national programs with private insurance (first voluntary, then mandatory) before turning to broader, general revenue-financed programs.[124]

Either an exclusively public or a public-private plan would have to establish national standards for benefits to be provided, maximum cost sharing that could be charged, quality assurance mechanisms, and hospital and physician rates (similar to state rate-setting programs). The concept of uniform national fees was anathema only a few years ago but is now becoming accepted: Medicare already has a prospective payment system for hospitals, and there is serious talk of a Medicare fee schedule for physicians. The poor and people who are not attached to the workforce would be publicly subsidized in a uniform national program. The program could be administered by federal agencies or by states under federal contract with some flexibility to select providers, especially for the poor, employ cost-containment strategies, or encourage the development of cost-effective provider arrangements.

Despite the advantages of a uniform national program, its disadvantages are many. The United States is a very large country for such a system; the national government cannot always be sensitive to regional and local differences and needs. Yet if the national government delegates authority to states or fiscal agents, consistent and equitable administration would be difficult, as Medicare experience has shown.

A Federal Health Care Financing Program

Because of the weaknesses of a uniform national system and concerns about its political viability, some proponents of a national approach are urging a federalized system similar to Canada's.[2] They argue that the United States has moved away from centralized government administration in recent years, and states have evolved greater cost-containment and administrative skills. They also note the ability of state governments to respond to local needs and the value of flexibility to try a variety of payment methods, quality assurance systems, and delivery approaches. They point, for instance, to the various delivery systems that have emerged, reflecting the fertility of regional experimentation and evolution.

Under a federalized program each state would be required to assure that all its residents had health insurance meeting certain minimum federal standards. Such a mandate on states would be enforced through either the offer of an adequate national financing share (as is done in Canada) or the threat of withholding other federal funds. States have balked at the latter strategy in enforcing the 55-mile per hour speed limit, raising the drinking age, or achieving Clean Air Act goals. The former strategy managed to bring all states but Arizona into Medicaid within that program's first 3 years and therefore appears to be a more productive incentive.

The federalized model could allow states considerable latitude in determining how to achieve universal protection, for instance through mandates on employers plus public financing for the unemployed and/or public institutions or alternatively through a totally public program financed by income, payroll, or excise taxes. It need not follow the Canadian model of publicly financed insurance.* The variety of possible systems is demonstrated by current experiments in several states. In spring 1988, Massachusetts enacted an

---

*Canada's system is often held up as a useful model for the United States, partially because of a presumed similar western tradition and because physicians and hospitals are paid on a fee-for-service basis in both countries. There are, however, a number of important differences between Canada and the United States. Private health insurance for basic medical care is prohibited in Canada, and the insurance industry apparently had little political ability to forestall its extinction. Furthermore, in Canada there are no HMOs or other arrangements whereby physicians share financial risk. Like all public systems, Canada's has waiting lists for some elective procedures, a fact of life that the population endures, but with which Americans might be less patient.

employer-based insurance program for workers with a publicly funded program for other residents. The state of Washington is testing a prepaid insurance program for low-income residents. Arizona is attempting to offer its AHCCCS program to small employers to extend workplace insurance. Wisconsin is designing a statewide health insurance program through which competing prepaid health plans would be available to employees of private employers as well as to government employees and public beneficiaries. Conceptually, its program is designed to assure that all the state's residents have basic health insurance through relatively comprehensive, organized delivery systems. A bill in California would require all employers to provide employee insurance and would cover the poor through publicly funded programs.[125] In a federalized system that authorizes differences among states, wealthier states would offer or require more benefits than other states, as occurs to some extent in Canada.* This may be a small price to pay for flexibility and the ability to respond to local needs.

Opposition to a federalized national financing system will come from two camps: people who oppose any national health plan (employers forced to provide mandated benefits, providers perceiving their incomes will suffer, insurers whose roles may be diminished, and opponents of any increased taxation or government role in health programs) and people who prefer a uniform approach. The latter camp will raise concerns about persistent variations among states and may also challenge the ability and willingness of state governments to administer a complex system. Certainly, some states have proven themselves better able and more willing than others to operate their Medicaid programs with sensitivity and creativity.[59] In addition to sharing in financing, an important role for the federal government in a federalized insurance program would be to monitor states' performance so that all U.S. citizens would have access to basic medical care.

Although a broad-based publicly financed health program for all Americans is a worthy goal, it may be irresponsible to reject short-term, less comprehensive solutions. It must be remembered,

---

*Coverage of some services, such as long-term care, varies among provinces. Although primary care is widely available, high-technology medicine is not as accessible, because government budget limits have forced provinces and providers explicitly to ration some kinds of equipment and new tertiary care resources.[126]

for instance, that in 1974 advocates of the publicly financed Health Security Act opposed the private insurance mandate of the Kennedy-Mills legislation,[2] holding out for something better; these forces lost the momentum for a national health care financing program that might have produced a reasonable, if imperfect, solution.

Public Support for a National Health Plan

Public opinion polls show increasing support for some type of national health care financing program, although perhaps under a less politically charged rubric than "national health insurance." For instance, in a recent referendum Massachusetts voters by a 2-to-1 margin urged the U.S. Congress "to enact a national health program" that provides universal coverage, is equitably financed and efficient, and costs no more than the previous year's share of the GNP devoted to health care.[127] A series of national Roper polls showed that although in 1982 only 44% of respondents felt that the government should make a major effort to set up "a national health insurance system for all citizens," by 1984, 53% supported such a statement.[128] In a 1983 Roper poll, however, 49% of the respondents preferred the "present system of private health plans," compared with only 41% who favored "a national insurance plan provided through the government."[128] This sentiment contrasts somewhat with a national *New York Times* poll in 1982, wherein 48% reported favoring a tax-supported government insurance plan.[128]

A plurality of respondents to a 1982 *Time* magazine poll strongly preferred to see medical care and poverty programs run by the states, rather than the federal government.[128] Thus, a federalized approach would probably have more popular support than a centralized or uniform national program.

These national polls apparently did not ask Americans whether they would willingly pay higher taxes to finance a publicly supported health plan. But a 1983 survey conducted by the Colorado Hospital Association found that 63% of respondents preferred increased taxes to reduced health care programs for the poor (in contrast, 60% favored defense spending cuts rather than tax increases for defense). To pay for unsponsored hospital patients, half the respondents favored increased taxes; only 23% preferred higher insurance premiums (cost shifting).[129] Recent polls in Missouri also showed that 56% of residents would support a sales tax and 33% would support an income tax surcharge to finance medical care for the uninsured.*

Costs of and Revenue Sources for a National Health Plan

Opponents of any national health care plan will surely raise concerns about cost containment. Ironically, as both overall and per capita medical care expenditures continue to rise faster than the growth in the general United States economy, and in view of the success of national systems such as Canada's in restraining this escalation, cost control through fixed government budgets, leading to provider fee schedules and risk-sharing contracts, may actually be the major argument in favor of a national health care financing program. In the short term, the nation's budget deficit makes unlikely a substantial new federal financial commitment. However, a program could be phased in by type of service or age group.[2] Canada enacted hospital insurance 10 years before physician insurance (although this may explain why physicians who make hospitalization decisions are not placed at risk for overall health costs through prepaid HMO-type arrangements). Medicaid expansion has encouraged phasing in coverage of children, and this approach could be used for currently uncovered groups, especially those dependent on public funds.

Several potential revenue sources exist for the publicly funded portions of a national health care financing program. Income taxes, the most progressive and efficient form of taxation, especially at the federal level, could be used. Taxes on insurance premiums, now in place in many states, institutionalize the current cost shift by burdening purchasers of health insurance but are somewhat progressive because both employer contributions and total premiums increase with family income.[84] To be equitable and not counterproductive, however, premium taxes would have to apply to self-insured firms as well as insurance carriers. Payroll taxes, though often used for financing employee benefits, have the disadvantage of making labor expensive, especially relative to foreign labor mar-

---

*Personal communication, Jerry Burch, Missouri House of Representatives.

kets.[130] Excise taxes are another source of revenue for state or federal governments. Imposing a sales tax on hospital revenues further sanctions current cost shifting but may be more politically feasible in the short run than other new revenue measures. Increasing alcohol and tobacco taxes is frequently justified because consumers of such products have greater health care needs than other groups. Excise taxes, especially on products used disproportionately by the poor, are, however, regressive. Although among the most politically viable of the new taxes, such excise taxes are more appropriate as a deterrent to unhealthy behavior than as a means of financing medical care for the uninsured.

Conclusion

A national strategy for access to medical care can take a number of directions, from modestly encouraging states and employers to increase insurance coverage to mandating a federalized, uniform, or even centralized public or public-private system. Because imperatives and priorities will change with the vagaries of the political process, what is important today is not the specific system formulation but federal leadership on this issue. The national government, both Congress and the Executive Branch, must acknowledge that access to medical care for the poor and uninsured is a national problem. HHS Secretary Bowen is to be commended for initiating this discussion, albeit with a fairly narrow focus on some of the catastrophic health care needs of the elderly. As Fein suggested, the debate must begin by developing agreement on principles by which any program can be judged.[2]

The dilemma facing policy makers is how to reconcile apparently broad public support for equality of access with our free-market preference for health care production and distribution—"egalitarian distribution and libertarian production" (p. 27).[1] Public acceptance of the need for a national health plan seems to be increasing, but the nation's schizophrenia over improving access while preserving private delivery and payment systems, and its nervousness about new taxes, mirrors the debate among policy makers and legislators. Achieving a consensus will not be easy.

Americans will disagree on specific solutions, but we must begin the discussion. A national strategy must lay out the entire policy solution, even though it undoubtedly must be phased in over time. At a minimum it must specify the timetable and the public and private sector responsibilities to turn policy into reality. If the nation does not put access to medical care on its agenda and if the number of uninsured people and medical care expenditures both continue to increase, by the end of this century the polls will show much greater support for a national health plan.

Meanwhile, the nation can take initial steps to increase protection for the poor gradually. If the proportion of uninsured people stabilizes, society can more easily afford to help them. If the proportion does not stabilize, however, failing to assist the uninsured will jeopardize the stability of our entire society. Fragmentary solutions addressing the greatest or most vocal needs will confine the problem in the short term, but only a long-term strategy holds promise for controlling medical care expenditures and for assuring equitable access to needed care for all Americans. A civilized society should do no less.

References

1. Reinhardt U. Health care for America's poor: The economics of a hot potato. Princeton Alum Weekly 1985;25–29.

2. Fein R. Medical care, medical costs. Cambridge, MA: Harvard University Press, 1986.

3. Robert Wood Johnson Foundation. Special Report, Access to health care in the United States: Results of a 1986 survey. Princeton, NJ: Robert Wood Johnson Foundation, 1987.

4. Starfield B. Motherhood and apple pie: The effectiveness of medical care for children. Milbank Mem Fund Q 1985;63(3):523–546.

5. Hadley J. More medical care, better health? Washington DC: Urban Institute Press, 1982.

6. Berki SE. A look at catastrophic medical expenses and the poor. Health Affairs 1986;5(4):138–145.

7. Cummings HK, Smith JP. Financing indigent care: Public problems and private responsibilities. Fed Amer Hosp Review 1985;52–54.

8. Himmelstein D et al. Patient transfers: Medical practice as social triage. Am J Public Health 1984;74(5):494–497.

9. Ansell D, Schiff R. Patient dumping. JAMA 1987;257(11):1500–1502.

10. U.S. House of Representatives Committee on Government Operations. Equal access to health care: Patient dumping. House Report 100–531, Washington, DC, March 25, 1988.

11. Aday L, Andersen R. National profile of access to medical care: Where do we stand? Am J Public Health 1984;74(12):1331–1339.

12. Andersen R. Health status indices and access to medical care. Am J Public Health 1978;68(5):458–463.

13. Freeman HE, Blendon RJ, Aiken LH, Sudman S, Mullinex CF, Corey CR. Americans report on their access to health care. Health Affairs 1987;6(1):6–18.

14. Institute of Medicine. Preventing low birthweight. Washington, DC: National Academy Press, 1985.

15. Logan A, Milne B, Achber C, Campbell W, Haynes R. Cost-effectiveness of a worksite hypertension treatment program. Hypertention 1981;3(2):211–218.

16. President's Commission for the Study of Ethical Problems in Medicine and Biomedical and Behavioral Research. Securing access to health care. Volume 1. Washington, DC: U.S. Superintendent of Documents, 1983.

17. Institute of Medicine. Health care in a context of civil rights. Washington, DC: National Academy Press, 1981.

18. Andersen R, Chen M, Aday L, Cornelius L. Health status and medical care utilization. Health Affairs 1987;6(1):136–156.

19. Davis K, Schoen K. Health and the war on poverty. Washington, DC: Brookings Institution, 1978.

20. Termination from Medi-Cal: Does it affect health? N Engl J Med 1984;311(7):480–484.

21. Wilensky GR, Walden DC, Kasper JA. The uninsured and their use of health services. Hyattsville, MD: National Center for Health Services Research, 1981.

22. Colorado Task Force on the Medically Indigent. Colorado's sick and uninsured—We can do better. Denver: Piton Foundation, 1984.

23. Berk ML, Taylor AK. Women and divorce: Health insurance coverage, utilization, and health care expenditures. Am J Public Health 1984;74(11):1276–1278.

24. Kasper JA, Walden DC, Wilensky GR. Who are the uninsured? Data preview 1. Hyattsville, MD: National Center for Health Services Research, US-DHHS, 1980.

25. Monheit AC, Hagan MM, Berk ML, Farley PJ. The employed uninsured and the role of public policy. Inquiry 1985;22:348–364.

26. Taylor AK, Lawson WR. Employer and employee expenditures for private health insurance. Data preview 7. Hyattsville, MD: National Center for Health Services Research, USDHHS, 1981.

27. U.S. Small Business Administration Office of Advocacy. Small business and health care: Providing affordable benefits. Washington, DC: U.S. Small Business Administration, 1986.

28. Farley P. Private health insurance in the United States. Data preview 23. Rockville, MD: National Center for Health Services Research, USDHHS, 1986.

29. Moyer ME, Cahill JA. HHS survey illustrates difference in large, small employers' health plans. Business & Health 1984;1(10):50–51.

30. Boulder County Task Force on Health Care Access. Improving access to health care in Boulder County: Assessing community needs. Boulder, CO: Boulder County Community Action Programs, 1986.

31. Luehrs J, Desonia R. A review of state task forces and special study recommendations to address health care for the indigent. Washington, DC: Intergovernmental Health Policy Project, 1984.

32. Rodat J. New Yorkers are losing their health insurance. Albany, NY: Signal Health, 1986.

33. Rhode Island Department of Health. Health care for the uninsured program proposal. Providence, RI: Rhode Island Dept of Health, 1986.

34. Davis K, Rowland D. Uninsured and underserved: Inequities in health care in the United States. Milbank Mem Fund Q 1983;61(2):149–176.

35. Wilensky GR, Farley PJ, Taylor AK. Variations in health insurance coverage: Benefits vs. premiums. Milbank Mem Fund Q 1984;62(1):53–81.

36. Wilensky GR. Data watch: Health care, the poor, and the role of Medicaid. Health Affairs 1982;1(4):93–100.

37. Newacheck P, Halfon N. Access to ambulatory care services for economically disadvantaged children. Pediatrics 1986;78(5):813–819.

38. Davis K, Rowland D. Medicare policy. Baltimore: Johns Hopkins University Press, 1986.

39. Commission on Elderly People Living Alone. Medicare's poor. New York: Commonwealth Fund, 1987.

40. Farley PJ. Who are the underinsured? Milbank Mem Fund Q 1985;63(3):476–503.

41. Blendon R, Rogers D. Cutting Medical care costs. JAMA 1983;250(14):1880–1885.

42. Starfield B. Family income, ill health, and medical care of U.S. children. J Pub Health Policy 1982;3(3):244–259.

43. National Center for Health Statistics. Monthly vital statistics report 1986;35(6).

44. Andersen R, Aday L, Lyttle C, Llewellyn C, Meei-Shia C. Ambulatory care and insurance coverage in an era of constraint. Chicago: Pluribus Press, 1987.

45. Congressional Budget Office. Catastrophic medical expenses: Patterns in the non-elderly, non-poor population. Washington, DC: Congressional Budget Office, 1982.

46. Blumenthal D. The social responsibility of physicians in a changing health care system. Inquiry 1986;23(3):268–274.

47. Feder J, Hadley J, Mullner R. Poor people and poor hospitals: Implications for public policy. J Health Polit Policy Law 1984;9(2):237–250.

48. Waldo D, Levit K, Lazenby H. National health expenditures 1985. Health Care Financ Rev 1986;8(1):1–22.

49. Eby CL, Cohodes DR. What do we know about rate-setting? J Health Polit Policy Law 1985;10(2):299–327.

50. Feldstein PJ. Health care economics. New York: John Wiley, 1983.

51. Merrill J. Competition vs. regulation: Some empirical evidence. J Health Polit Policy Law 1986;10(4):613–623.

52. Butler P. Legal problems in Medicaid. In: Roemer R, McKray G, eds. Legal aspects of health policy. Westport, CT: Greenwood Press; 1980:215–241.

53. Kerr-Mills Program of Health Care for the Aged, P.L. 86–778, 74 Stat. 987 (1060).

54. Freeman H, Kirkmann-Liff B. Health care under AHCCCS: An examination of Arizona's alternative to Medicaid. Health Serv Res 1985;20(3):245–266.

55. U.S. General Accounting Office. An evaluation of 1981 AFDC changes— Final report. Washington, DC: U.S. General Accounting Office, 1985.

56. Rosenbaum S, Johnson K. Providing health care for low income children: Reconciling child health goals with child health financing realities. Milbank Mem Fund Q 1986;64(3):442–478.

57. Summary of state disproportionate share provisions. Health advocate. Los Angeles: National Health Law Program, 1986.

58. Joe T, Meltzer J, Yu P. Arbitrary access to care: The case for reforming Medicaid. Health Affairs 1985;4(1):24–40.

59. Erdman K, Wolfe S. Poor health care for poor Americans: A ranking of state Medicaid programs. Washington, DC: Public Citizen Health Research Group, 1987.

60. American Hospital Association Special Committee on Care for the Indigent. Cost and compassion—Recommendations for avoiding a crisis in care for the medically indigent. Chicago: American Hospital Association, 1986.

61. Health Care Financing Administration. Health care financing program statistics, Medicare and Medicaid data book 1984. Baltimore: HCFA, 1986.

62. Mitchell JB, Cromwell J. Access to private physicians for public patients: Participation in Medicaid and Medicare. In: Securing access to health care. Volume 3. President's Commission for the Study of Ethical Problems in Medicine and Biomedical and Behavioral Research. Washington, DC: U.S. Government Printing Office, 1983.

63. National Study Group on State Medicaid Strategies. Restructuring Medicaid: An agenda for change. Washington, DC: Center for the Study of Social Change, 1983.

64. U.S. Census Bureau. Money income and poverty status of family persons in the U.S. 1985. Series P-60-154. Washington, DC: U.S. Census Bureau, 1986.

65. Butler P. Legal obligations of state and local governments for indigent health care. In: Curtis R, ed. Access to care for the medically indigent: A resource document for state and local officials. Washington, DC: Academy for State and Local Government; 1985:13–44.

66. Abel P, Glazner J. Expenditures on health care and funds flow—Colorado and the United States, 1976–1982. Denver, CO: Colorado Department of Health, 1986.

67. Desonia R, King K. State programs of assistance for the medically indigent. Washington, DC: Intergovernmental Health Policy Project, 1985.

68. National Health Law Program. Manual on state and local government responsibilities to provide medical care for indigents. Los Angeles: National Health Law Program, 1985.

69. Bartlett L. State level policies and programs. In: Curtis R, ed. Access to care for the medically indigent: A resource document for state and local officials. Washington, DC: Academy for State and Local Government; 1985:54–72.

70. Feder J, Hadley J, Mullner R. Falling through the cracks: Poverty, insurance coverage, and hospital care for the poor, 1980 and 1982. Milbank Mem Fund Q 1984;62(4):544–566.

71. Lewin L, Lewin M. Financing charity care in an era of competition. Health Affairs 1987;6(1):47–60.

72. Dowell MA. Indigent access to hospital emergency room services. Clearinghouse Rev 1984;5:483–499.

73. Hospital Trustees of New York State. Risking the future. Albany: Hospital Trustees of New York State, 1987.

74. Utah County v. Intermountain Health Care, 709 P.2d 265 (Utah 1985).

75. Medical Center Hospital of Vermont v. City of Burlington, No.S-658-87CnC, Chittenden Superior Court, September 22, 1987.

76. Shonick W, Roemer R. Public hospitals under private management. Berkeley, CA: University of California Institute of Governmental Studies, 1983.

77. Starr P. The social transformation of American medicine. New York: Basic Books, 1982.

78. Colorado Task Force on the Medically Indigent. Background papers, vol. 3. Denver, CO: Piton Foundation, 1984.

79. Myers B. Public subsidies for hospital care for the poor. In: Sloan FA, ed. Uncompensated hospital care: Rights and responsibilities. Baltimore: Johns Hopkins University Press; 1986:126–147.

80. Vladeck B. How much indigent care should hospitals provide? Health Manage Q 1985:2–4.

81. Ohsfeldt R. Uncompensated medical services provided by physicians and hospitals. Med Care 1985;25:1338–1344.

82. Sloan FA, Valvona J, Mullner R. Identifying the issues: A statistical profile. In: Sloan FA, ed. Uncompensated hospital care: Rights and responsibilities. Baltimore: Johns Hopkins University Press; 1986:16–53.

83. Wilensky GR, Rossiter LF. The relative importance of physician-induced demand in the demand for medical care. Milbank Mem Fund Q 1983;61(2):252–277.

84. Wilensky GR. Solving uncompensated hospital care: Targeting the indigent and the uninsured. Health Affairs 1984;3(4):50–62.

85. Florida Task Force on Competition and Consumer Choice in Health Care. An opportunity for leadership. Tallahassee, FL: Office of the Governor, 1984.

86. Hadley J, Feder J. Hospital cost-shifting and care for the uninsured. Health Affairs 1984;4(3):67–80.

87. Dallek G, Hurwit C, Golde M. Insuring the uninsured: Options for state action. Washington, DC: National Health Care Campaign, 1988.

88. Wilensky G, Ladenheim K. The uninsured: Response and responsibility. Frontiers of Health Services Management 1987;4(2):3–31.

89. Luft HS. Assessing the evidence on HMO performance. Milbank Mem Fund Q 1980;58(4):501–536.

90. Darling H. The role of the federal government in assuring access to health care. Inquiry 1986;23(3):286–298.

91. Swartz K. Changes in the noninstitutionalized Medicaid population, 1979–1983. Washington, DC: Urban Institute Working Paper, 1987.

92. Southern Regional Task Force on Infant Mortality. A fiscal imperative: Prenatal and infant care. Washington, DC: Southern Governors' Association, 1985.

93. Hill-Burton Hospital Construction Act of 1946, 42 U.S.C. 291 et seq., P.L. 79-725 (1946).

94. Coker v. Hunt Memorial Hospital District, No. Ca-3-86-1200-H, N.D. Tex. July 29, 1986.

95. Governor's Commission on Ohio Health Care Costs. Final report. Columbus, OH: Office of the Governor, 1984.

96. Standard Oil of California v. Agsalud, 633 F.2d 760 (9th Cir. 1980), aff'd, 454 U.S. 801 (1982); Metropolitan Life Insurance Co. v. Massachusetts, 53 U.S.L.W. 4616 (1985).

97. O'Brien R, Kaufman S. A model multiple employer trust expands small business health benefits options. Business and Health 1984;1(6):47.

98. American Hospital Association. Promoting health insurance in the workplace: State and local initiatives to increase private coverage. Chicago: American Hospital Association, 1988.

99. Health Care for the Uninsured Program. Quarterly report (1). Washington, DC: Alpha Center, December 1986.

100. Health Care for the Uninsured Program. Quarterly report (2). Washington, DC: Alpha Center, March 1987.

101. Bovberg R. Insuring the uninsured through private action: Ideas and initiatives. Inquiry 1986;23(4):403–418.

102. Bradbury R. Can competition and choice serve the needs of the under- and uninsured? Health Manage Q 1985:12–15.

103. Lewin L, Lewin M. Health care for the uninsured. Business & Health 1984;1(9):9–14.

104. Wilensky G. Testimony before Subcommittee on Intergovernmental Relations, Committee on Governmental Affairs, Hearing on Access to Health Insurance and Health Care. Washington, DC: U.S. Senate Hearing No. 99–760; 1986.

105. Ethridge L. Ethics and the new insurance market. Inquiry 1986;23(3):308–315.

106. Lohr K. Use of medical care in the Rand health insurance experiment. Med Care 1986;24(a) (Supplement).

107. Neuschler E. Alternative financing and delivery systems: Managed health care. In: Curtis R, Hill I, eds. Affording access to quality care. Washington, DC: National Governors' Association; 1986:201–242.

108. Kirkmann-Liff B, Christianson C, Kirkmann-Liff T. The evaluation of Arizona's indigent health care system. Health Affairs 1987;6(4):46–58.

109. Kirkmann-Liff B. Refusal of care: Evidence from Arizona. Health Affairs 1985;4(4):15–24.

110. Chavkin D, Tresseder A. California's prepaid health plan program: Can the patient be saved? Hastings Law J 1977;28(3):685–760.

111. Internal Revenue Code Section 106, 26 U.S. Code 106.

112. Internal Revenue Code Section 105, 26 U.S. Code 105.

113. Enthoven A. A new proposal to reform the tax treatment of health insurance. Health Affairs 1984;3(1):21–39.

114. Internal Revenue Code Section 162, 26 U.S. Code 162.

115. Employee costs—Keeping them in line without stepping on the staff. Med Econ 1987;64(22):117–127.

116. Brook R. Does free care improve adults' health? N Engl J Med 1983;309(23):1426–1433.

117. Eastern Kentucky Welfare Rights Organization v. Simon, 426 U.S. 26 (1976).

118. Rose M. The Internal Revenue Service's "contribution" to the health problems of the poor. Catholic Law Review 1971;21(1):35–62.

119. Van Steenwick J. Evaluation of the impact of Hawaii's mandatory health insurance law. New York: Martin E. Segal Co., 1978.

120. Curtis R. The role of state governments in assuring access to health care. Inquiry 1986;23(3):277–285.

121. Congressional Budget Office. Medicaid: Choices for 1982 and beyond. Washington, DC: Congressional Budget Office, 1981.

122. Meiners M. The case for long-term care insurance. Health Affairs 1983;2(2):55–79.

123. Feder J, Moon M, Scanlon W. Medicare reform: Nibbling at catastrophic costs. Health Affairs 1987;6(4):5–19.

124. Roemer M. National strategies for health care organization. Ann Arbor, MI: Health Administration Press, 1985.

125. Task Force on State Health Insurance as Part of a National Health Program: Report to the APHA Executive Board. Washington, DC: American Public Health Association, 1988.

126. Igelhart J. Canada's health care system. N Engl J Med 1986;315:778–784.

127. Danielson D, Mazer A. Results of the Massachusetts referendum for a national health program. J Public Health Policy 1987;8(1):28–35.

128. Sherlock DB. Indigent care in rational markets. Inquiry 1986;23(3):261–267.

129. SRI Research Center. Colorado Hospital Association statewide opinion study. Lincoln, NE: SRI Research Center, 1983.

130. Thorow L. A bad idea for America. Boston Globe. 1987 Aug 25.

Appendix A
Sources of Data

The National Medical Care Expenditures Survey (NMCES) was an 18-month assessment of more than 14,000 families. Each family was interviewed in person five times in 1977 and 1978. The survey also gathered data from employers, health care providers, and insurance policies. It chronicled family experiences with health insurance coverage, health status, use of health care services, health care charges and payments, and sources of payment. Because it did not survey people who were institutionalized, it omitted the many Medicaid residents of nursing homes.

NMCES revealed that in early 1977, 12.6% of Americans had neither public nor private insurance, but, by its longitudinal design, it was able also to show fluctuating patterns of coverage: More than 8% of the population was uninsured during the entire year, and at least another 7% was uninsured part of the year, so about 16% of the population—over one-quarter more than the point-in-time estimate—lacked coverage during at least part of the year.[1] A 1983 survey of poor and near-poor people in Colorado revealed a similar pattern: 38% of the lower income population was uninsured at the time of the study, and 46% had been uninsured all or part of the previous year.[2]

Analysis of health care use shows that people who sometimes have health care insurance use health care differently when they are insured than when they are uninsured: When they are insured, their use is similar to that of people who are always insured, whereas their use when they are uninsured is similar to that of people who are always uninsured.[3] Insurance patterns over time are important to understand because fluctuations in insurance coverage change both the way health care is used and the likelihood that a person will face barriers to medical care. Most national and state studies describe the number of uninsured people at one specific time, but NMCES shows that the actual population at risk of facing access barriers during a given year may be much larger than point-in-time figures. For instance, in 1977, 26.7 million persons were uninsured at one point in the year;[1] but 18 million were uninsured during the entire year and 16 million were uninsured during a part of that year,[3] for a total of 34 million without insurance for at least part of the year.

NMCES provides a wealth of information on health care use and insurance coverage, but its 1977 data are criticized for being outdated, particularly in terms of the types of insurance policies available (employment-based benefits have changed in the past 10 years) and the size of the uninsured population. Because it was conducted before the most recent recession, NMCES is less likely to reflect current conditions affecting insurance status. The 1980 National Medical Care Utilization and Expenditure Survey (NMCUES) provides more recent data on the numbers of uninsured people and their use of services but not on the breadth of their coverage. More recent surveys suggest that the uninsured portion of the U.S. population may be rising. Despite its limitations, NMCES is useful to illustrate detailed characteristics of the uninsured and insured populations. Health status and patterns of health care use of these groups have probably not changed substantially since 1978, although as consumer cost sharing in health insurance increases, use of health care among the privately insured is likely to decline.[4]

A more current and regular source of data on the uninsured is the Current Population Survey (CPS) of the U.S. Census Bureau. Each March the Census Bureau collects demographic data through in-person surveys of a representative sample of Americans. Since 1979, CPS has included a set of questions on insurance coverage. It is a good source of data on demographic characteristics of the uninsured (although, like NMCES, it excludes institutionalized people), and it has the advantage of being fairly up-to-date. Because the questions about insurance have been asked for several years, CPS provides useful trend information. However, it reports respondents' recollections of their insurance experience for the previous year. Katherine Swartz, the principal researcher using CPS data, thinks that recall may be limited and that the data are probably more accurate for the year of response rather than the year the survey is meant to reflect. Another limitation of CPS data is that their validity is less well checked than the validity of NMCES data. Furthermore, CPS data do not include changes in insurance status during the year and do not cover use of health care or payment for care. Trend information from CPS can, however, be usefully combined with NMCES data on changes in insurance status, use of health care, and costs of health care to draw a broad composite picture of the uninsured.

Another source of health insurance data is the Survey of Income and Program Participation (SIPP), conducted quarterly by the Census Bureau since 1983. Like CPS, SIPP surveys respondents' demographic characteristics and health insurance status but does not cover use of health care or payment. Because SIPP is conducted more frequently than CPS and has a shorter recall period, its data may be more current than CPS data. But because it draws one annual sample, and experiences attrition among low-income respondents, it may underrepresent the poor over the course of a year.

References

1. Kasper JA, Walden DC, Wilensky GR. Who are the uninsured? Data preview 1. Hyattsville, MD: National Center for Health Services Research; 1980.

2. Colorado Task Force on the Medically Indigent. Colorado's sick and uninsured—We can do better. Denver, CO: Piton Foundation; 1983.

3. Wilensky GR, Walden DC, Kasper JA. The uninsured and their use of health services. Hyattsville, MD: National Center for Health Services Research; 1981.

4. Brook R. Does free care improve adults' health? N Engl J Med 1983; 309(23):1426–1433.

Appendix B
Characteristics of Patients Accounting for Uncompensated Hospital Care

Although uncompensated hospital care is not the primary focus of this analysis, it represents an important source of health care for the poor and uninsured. To understand who is receiving institutional charity, it is useful to examine data on the types of patients who receive uncompensated hospital care. Unfortunately, because of problems with definitions and data collection, there is little information available about the patients represented by "charity care" and hospital "bad debt." National data are collected by payer source, such as private insurance, Medicaid, Medicare, or "self-pay," a category into which hospitals place people with no insurance.

An Urban Institute study indicated that in 1980 uninsured self-pay patients accounted for 67% of hospital bad debt (the other 33% came from unpaid deductibles and coinsurance from Medicare, Blue Cross, and commercial insurers).[1] It is therefore assumed that the

107

characteristics of self-pay patients fairly accurately represent those of charity and bad debt patients. Data from the 1981 Hospital Discharge Survey of the National Center for Health Statistics include diagnoses and procedures provided to patients whose primary source of payment was listed as self-pay. These patients tended to receive routine care, not extraordinary or heroic medicine. More than 40% of self-pay patients were maternity cases: 39.7% were deliveries, and 4.8% were complications in pregnancy. Combined with accident cases (12.8% of self-pay patients), these categories accounted for more than half of the self-pay patients and 44% of the charges. Obstetrics and reproductive organ surgery accounted for more than half of the surgical cases and 40% of the surgical charges. The self-pay patients were more likely to have deliveries than were people insured by Medicaid or private insurance.[2,3]

Although self-pay patients contribute to hospital bad debt, not all fail to pay for their care. About 30% of self-pay charges are not collected, but national data do not permit analysis of the diagnoses of or services used by the self-pay patients who do not pay. It may be, for instance, that a large share of normal deliveries fall in the self-pay category because women of child-bearing age are less likely to be insured and because even insured patients are often not covered for this service.*

A study of the characteristics of patients assigned bad debt or charity care status in one Boulder County hospital shows that although obstetrical care was given in almost 40% of inpatient bad debt and charity cases, medical/surgical care was provided to more than 50% of these cases and cardiac and intensive care was given in the remainder.[4] This study also revealed differences among inpatients and emergency room users: Inpatients were more likely to be female, married, and from 19 to 25 years old, whereas emergency room users tended to be male, single, and 26 to 40 years old. Most of the patients assigned to charity and bad debt status were uninsured but employed, often in hotels, restaurants, or service firms.

---

*Title VII of the federal Civil Rights Law prohibits employers from sexual discrimination in health benefits. Thus, if firms offer hospitalization benefits, they cannot refuse to cover the costs of a normal delivery. However, firms with fewer than 15 empoyees are not subject to this requirement. 42 U.S.Code 2000e(b), 2000e(a)(1), 29 C.F.R.1604, App.

A 1987 study of self-pay and charity patients in New York hospitals found that although these patients were less likely than other patients to be admitted to hospitals, once hospitalized they had longer lengths of stay for most conditions other than deliveries, substance abuse, mental illness, and injuries.[5] These differences persisted among all age groups. Because there would be financially no incentive to hospitalize uninsured people excessively, such longer lengths of stay suggest that self-pay and charity patients may be sicker than other patients on admission, perhaps because of delays in seeking care.

It would be useful to know more about the patients who account for hospital bad debt and charity care. For instance, do they obtain appropriate care at early stages of illness, or do they delay care until health problems become more costly and difficult to treat? As hospitals reexamine their charity care policies, characteristics of the patients responsible for uncompensated care cases may be further investigated, which will more fully define this portion of the uninsured population.

References

1. Mullstein S. The uninsured and the financing of uncompensated care: Scope, costs, and policy options. Inquiry 1984;21:214–229.

2. Sloan FA, Valvona J, Mullner R. Identifying the issues: A statistical profile. In: Sloan FA, ed. Uncompensated hospital care: Rights and responsibilities. Baltimore: Johns Hopkins University Press; 1986:16–53.

3. Sloan FA, Morrisey MA, Valvona J. Hospital care for the"self-pay" patient. J Health Polit Policy Law 1988;13(1):83–102.

4. Boulder County Task Force on Health Care Access. Improving access to health care in Boulder County: Assessing community needs. Boulder, CO: Boulder County Community Action Programs; 1986.

5. Hospital Trustees of New York State. Risking the future. Albany, NY: Hospital Trustees of New York State; 1987.

Patricia A. Butler, JD, has been an Associate Director of the National Health Law Program and Staff Director of the Colorado Task Force on the Medically Indigent. She has also served as Chair of the APHA Task Force on State Health Insurance as Part of a National Health Program and is a member of the Robert Wood Johnson Foundation's National Advisory Committee on its Health Care for the Uninsured Initiative. She is currently a health policy consultant in Boulder, Colorado, and has acted as consultant to the National Governors' Association, the National Conference of State Legislatures, the National Association of Counties, and several state governments.

0055170

TOO POOR TO BE SICK
ACCESS TO MED

BUTLER